EVERYTHING

YOU NEED TO KNOW ABOUT...

YOGA

EVERYTHING

YOU NEED TO KNOW ABOUT...

YOGA

CYNTHIA WORBY MSW, MPH, RYT

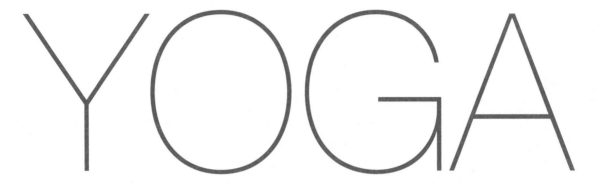

David & Charles

A DAVID & CHARLES BOOK

David & Charles is a subsidiary of F&W (UK) Ltd.,

an F&W Publications Inc. company

First published in the UK in 2004

First published in the USA as The Everything® Yoga Book,

by Adams Media Corporation in 2002

Project Manager Ian Kearey

Cover Design Ali Myer

A catalogue record for this book is available from the British Library.

ISBN 0 7153 1952 3

Printed in Great Britain by CPI Bath

for David & Charles

Brunel House   Newton Abbot   Devon

Visit our website at www.davidandcharles.co.uk

David & Charles books are available from all good bookshops;

alternatively you can contact our Orderline on (0)1626 334555

or write to us at FREEPOST EX2110, David & Charles Direct,

Newton Abbot, TQ12 4ZZ (no stamp required UK mainland).

Contents

Dedication

To my mother, who loved writing and instilled in me a love of the written word, and to my father, from whom I inherited a voracious love of reading.

Acknowledgments

There are countless people who directly and indirectly have contributed to this book. I want to thank all my family and friends, for their love, support and the ability to listen, as well as the many students over the years who have also been my teachers. So many thanks go to Gloria DeMarchis, a wonderful therapist and friend, who started me on the path to wholeness, suggested I try yoga many years ago, and guided me through a difficult time in my life. Thank you to Pam Hogan, whose wisdom and guidance have been invaluable. A big thank-you to my first yoga teacher, Tao Porchon Lynch, who inspired me and sparked my love of yoga, and who encouraged me to start teaching. Thank you to Nevine Michaan, who generously shared her unique style of teaching yoga, to Beryl Bender Birch and Thom Birch, who opened up their home and their hearts while teaching teachers how to teach Ashtanga (Power Yoga), and to Mary Dunn, senior Iyengar teacher, who beautifully teaches the fine art, science and philosophy of Iyengar Yoga.

A big thank-you goes to Sara Rubin, for giving literary agent June Clark my name as a good (yoga) person to write this book. And a thank-you to writer Eve Marx, who answered my questions (as a complete neophyte in the publishing world) about how to negotiate the book contract, and assured me that I was up to the task of writing this book. A very big thank-you to my agent, June Clark, for all her support and e-mails throughout the writing process, for helping me through my nervousness about beginning such an endeavour, and for finding Ron Rinaldi, our photographer. Thank you to Ron, for such beautiful, clear photographs. Thank you to my editors Pam Liflander and Bethany Brown at Adams Media.

I want to thank Monica Beatriz, good friend, fellow student and teacher on the path of yoga, for her invaluable friendship and insights and her willingness to be one of the yoga models in this book.

An enormously big thank-you goes to Mary Sinclair, intermediate Iyengar yoga teacher, who gave so generously of her time, knowledge and compassionate spirit as a teacher, and who, throughout the writing of this book, spent countless hours reading and editing the book with me (from a yogic perspective). In addition, Mary helped organize the photo shoot and virtually directed the shoot. She also modelled many of the beautiful postures in this book. Thank you, Mary, for your invaluable knowledge, creativity and insights.

Thank you to my Dad, who read the book as a layperson, to make sure that it could be understood by those unfamiliar with yoga.

A big, big thank-you to Joe Nero, who has given me so much love and support over the years and believes in me 100 per cent, and who put up with me during the writing of this book, when I was often literally consumed by the process.

My thank-yous would be incomplete if I didn't include my greatest teachers, my children Jess, Becca and Sam, who also show me understanding, love and support, among other things, every day of my life.

A last big thank-you to the vast lineage of yoga teachers who have shared their knowledge and helped yoga evolve throughout the ages.

Namaste.

Introduction

Yoga has been around for 5,000 years – and for a very good reason: It works. In the past 30 years or so, yoga has become increasingly popular in the United Kingdom and has entered the mainstream of public consciousness. Celebrities like Madonna, Sting and Geri Halliwell are seriously involved in yoga and praise its benefits highly. In the USA, Oprah Winfrey devoted an entire hour-long TV show to yoga, in which Rodney Yee, world-renowned and highly recognized yoga teacher, taught yoga to the studio audience; and model, Christy Turlington, herself an avid yogi, discussed her love of yoga and presented her line of yoga clothing called Nuala.

Newspaper and magazine articles on yoga abound. Health clubs include yoga classes on their schedules, and health insurance companies are recommending yoga therapy.

It certainly seems as if everyone is talking about yoga these days – or trying it. The british Wheel of Yoga estimates that there are as many as 500,000 people practising yoga regularly in the UK at the present time, while *Yoga Journal* recently estimated that one in 13 Americans had either tried or was thinking of trying yoga.

As a yoga teacher and student, I have observed the broad spectrum of people who are inquiring about yoga and taking classes. Yoga is no longer just for people from the Sixties generation, who burned incense, chanted and wore baggy trousers. And it is certainly not a fad! Writers, artists, teachers, housewives, stockbrokers, film producers, college students, lawyers, architects, retired people, carpenters and plumbers alike are all doing yoga.

So what is all the fuss about, and what can yoga do for you? Yoga can help you look and feel great, open and strengthen your body, quieten and focus your mind, relieve tension, increase your self-knowledge and awareness, improve your quality of life and change how you see the world. It has a profound and lasting effect on how you treat yourself and others. Time spent doing yoga is an opportunity to reconnect intimately with yourself on many levels and to give yourself your complete attention. When was the last time you did that? By practising yoga you can rejuvenate, care for and nurture yourself at the deepest levels, resulting in greater reservoirs of compassion and tolerance for other people and a positive impact on your relationships. Most importantly, you will develop a better relationship with yourself.

You will experience longer periods of calm and clarity. All those minor daily annoyances, emotional ups and downs and responsibilities will be brought into a broader perspective, which allows them to come and go without becoming too attached to you. You will begin to understand what is most life-affirming, beneficial, lasting and important to you.

Everything You Need to Know About Yoga is a general introduction that has a style, language and format that are easy to read and follow. The language of yoga is Sanskrit, an ancient and beautiful language. Sanskrit, with the English translation, will be used throughout the book, when appropriate. Please do not be intimidated by Sanskrit. It is a phonetic language, which sounds just as it is spelled, unlike our crazy English language. Of course, the Sanskrit alphabet is different from ours. But don't worry – I only include the English translation in this book. When you read the Sanskrit name of a pose, say it out loud, just as it is written, and you will be speaking Sanskrit!

The book contains information about what yoga is, its history and philosophy, the different styles of yoga, the health benefits of yoga, what you need to get started, yoga poses to practise, relaxation and meditation practices and yoga for specific needs, as well as yoga resources. The description of poses includes photographs illustrating the postures, as well as any useful modifications to the postures. Before you practise the postures, look at the pictures and read the description of how to do the poses, the ways to practise and any contraindications. It is my wish that this book will educate and motivate you to include yoga in your daily life.

CHAPTER 1

What Yoga Is

Although yoga has been around for thousands of years, many people still aren't quite sure what it is. If you count yourself in this group, you're not alone. This chapter spells out exactly what yoga is – dispelling myths and re-affirming thoughts along the way.

An Ancient Art and Science

Yoga is an ancient art and science from India, originally designed to strengthen and align the body and quieten and focus the mind for meditation. It has been successfully adapted to the needs and lifestyles of Westerners. Yoga is a teaching that is strongly grounded in physiological reality. Your experience of the world greatly depends upon the health of your nervous system, which is impacted on by environment, heredity and the foods you eat. The practices of yoga strengthen and purify the nervous system so we can most clearly perceive and interact in the world in a conscious and positive manner.

Most of the yoga practised in the West is what is known as *Hatha Yoga*. Hatha Yoga works with postures (known as *asana*), breathing techniques (known as *pranayama*), conscious relaxation (known as *pratyahara* and *dharana*) and meditation (known as *dhyana*).

The Uniting of Body, Mind and Spirit

The word *yoga* means, literally, 'to yoke or join'. In the practice of yoga, we join and integrate the mind, body and spirit into one aligned and cohesive unit. The body is the gross manifestation of spirit. Working with the body through yoga connects you with spirit, while unravelling the emotional, physical, and mental knots that bind you and blind you from your true nature. This process allows your essence to shine through and illuminate your entire being. It is a catalyst enabling you to grow in whatever way is natural and self-affirming.

Yoga is one of the oldest *holistic* health-care systems in existence, focusing on both the mind and the body. In the Western world, most people live in their heads more than in their bodies. The educational system is focused on book-learning; many jobs are either cerebral or entirely physical (few incorporate both). And Western medicine has traditionally focused almost solely on the physical aspect of health, neglecting the emotional and spiritual aspects that yoga attends to.

Through the practice of yoga postures and breath work, you can reconnect your body and mind and discover your spirit. You can become whole and regain an intimate knowledge of your real Self (not the little self with needs and wants that gnaw at you all day long). Yoga is the art of listening to all parts of your Self.

This ancient practice is a spiritual discipline with a code of ethics toward yourself and others. It is not a religion. It is a system for discovering and developing the true Self, an ancient method of psychotherapy (before there was one) and a potent self-evolutionary tool. In the classic text, *Yoga Sutra,* the spiritual path of yoga is laid out like a road map with discussion of the mental, physical and psychological benefits and roadblocks along the way.

 Each person has between 50,000 and 75,000 thoughts a day, and out of those thoughts at least 50,000 of them will be the same thoughts as he or she had yesterday. If you don't clean out the old thoughts to make room for the creation of new thoughts, it is difficult to process life's events, learn from them and progress.

A Language

Learning yoga is like learning a new language for your body and mind. Everyone knows that a language cannot be learned overnight. Yoga is a discipline that must be practised, refined and experienced. It is an experiential science in which you analyze your thoughts and actions. This is why yoga is described as a practice – you have to practise it to gain experience and self-knowledge from your efforts. It is a process that unfolds over time with trial and error, and one that cannot be rushed. Yoga helps develop patience and persistence.

Your body and mind are your laboratories of experimentation where useful patterns of thought and movement can develop and replace habitual patterns that are no longer appropriate. Many people begin yoga as a result of stress, inflexibility, poor posture or a condition that requires care.

A Powerful, Holistic and Transforming Tool

Yoga is also a powerful, holistic and transforming tool that calms and focuses the mind and develops innate intelligence and awareness. The postures, breath awareness and relaxation techniques develop your natural intuitive intelligence, and help your mind to focus on one thing at a time instead of jumping around like a hyperactive monkey. When the mind is focused, the nervous, circulatory and respiratory systems respond by slowing down. The body and mind start to relax. You feel calmer, think more clearly and feel centred and grounded. Over time, the mind and the intelligence are able to spread throughout the body, focusing on many points at one time. This is *meditation*.

As the mind quietens, the body opens to release unnecessary tension and long-held emotions. The emotions become balanced and moderate. The body develops balanced strength, and with strength comes flexibility and a stable core. You experience emotional equanimity and poise, like a tree that sways in the breeze but always comes back to the centre. Life will always have its sunny days and stormy times, but yoga creates a strong foundation with which you can endure life's unpredictable weather.

The yoga postures, known as *asanas,* have a very powerful effect on all systems of the body. Each asana is linked with the breath, which contains the life force or universal energy known as *prana.* Every inhalation brings prana and oxygen to all the cells in the body, and every exhalation releases toxins and waste.

A Therapeutic Tool

Yoga is also a therapeutic tool. Many ailments and disorders can be relieved by specific postures and breathing practices under the guidance of a qualified yoga teacher. Often people are amazed to find that their backaches, headaches and joint pain can disappear with regular practice. People with cancer, cardiac problems and multiple sclerosis can experience relief of some symptoms and develop the ability to relax more fully and cope with stress.

Something Everyone Can Do

Everyone can do yoga, regardless of age, size, flexibility or health. Many people unfamiliar with yoga think that they have to be like a bendy toy – able to touch their toes to their nose – but this is not true. Yoga is the great equalizer. Two people can walk into a yoga class, one very flexible with no strength and the other stiff (too strong) with little flexibility. The same poses done by these individuals will tighten up the overly flexible person and loosen the stiff person. Overweight people, pregnant women and older people can practise yoga and receive its benefits. There are many types of yoga suitable for anyone, and poses can *always* be modified to fit an individual's needs.

A Way to Have Fun

Yoga may sound like a lot of hard work, but it is also a lot of fun. Learning to move your body in new ways can make you feel very playful, like being a kid again! Going upside down in an inverted posture, such as a handstand, can be mood-elevating. Backbends are exhilarating and liberating. Although unfamiliar positions might bring up fears or feelings of 'I can't do that', once those feelings are conquered, feelings of mastery and accomplishment predominate, and you feel free, limitless and able to do anything! Yoga is all about exploration and being open to new ways of being. So find a class that suits you and have fun!

You may be eager to achieve the 'perfect' pose and correct bad postural habits. But it took a lifetime to get you where you are today. One yoga class won't change all that. In yoga, the journey is more important than the destination – and it's also a lot more interesting!

CHAPTER 2

What Yoga Can Do for You

People have been practising yoga for thousands of years because they get something out of it. In this chapter, you'll discover what that something is. When you practise yoga yourself, you'll see these benefits firsthand.

Renewed Energy

The yoga postures, known as *asanas,* bend the spine in many different ways:

· Forwards
· Backwards
· Side to side
· Twisting from one side to the other

Moving the spine in this way keeps the spine supple and healthy and nourishes the entire nervous system. The asanas release tension and blocked energy; lengthen and strengthen muscles; and tone, stimulate and massage the internal organs. As a result, the muscles and organs are bathed in blood, nutrients and prana. Every cell is rejuvenated and cleansed. Respiration, cardiac functioning, circulation, nervous system functioning, elimination and mental clarity improve. Fatigue and stress are reduced.

Next time you're feeling unhappily unattached, steal a look at the person on the yoga mat next to you. You could be looking at a potential partner who may share your love of yoga and philosophy of life. Just keep in mind that yoga should be an *inner*-directed experience. The most important thing is finding truth and happiness within yourself.

Energy to Age Gracefully

Yoga postures are anti-ageing and anti-gravity – they reduce the sagging of organs and muscles due to ageing and gravity's constant pull. The saying 'You're as young as your spine' is absolutely true. Regular practice of yoga postures maintains the suppleness and youth of the spine. The postures also develop coordination and balance – essential as one ages, for preventing falls. They improve posture and increase knowledge of body mechanics.

As people grow older, as life slows down a bit and as their responsibilities change, the desire to go inward and contemplate life grows. The system of yoga provides a wonderful framework for that inward search and growth. Conscious relaxation and meditation are time-tested tools for contemplation and inner wisdom.

Mary Pullig Schatz, MD, an American pathologist and yoga therapist, says that regular practice of Hatha Yoga can help maintain or restore muscle strength and adaptability, circulatory and respiratory efficiency, bone strength, sensitivity to insulin, normal bowel function, immune function, your ability to respond well to challenges and stress, and healthy lipid and cholesterol metabolism, among other things.

Staying Fit

Yoga is a wonderful way to get into shape. The postures tone organs and develop long, lean muscles. The practice of forward bends, back bends, lateral poses, twists and inversions balances and works every muscle, bone, joint and organ in the body. Weight-bearing yoga poses, crucial for healthy bones, provide one of the best exercise systems known to man. Flexibility and strength of the muscles and range of motion in the joints greatly increase. Stamina and endurance also improve.

Improved Circulation

Yoga postures promote better circulation of blood and lymph throughout the body. Inversions such as the headstand and shoulderstand reverse the flow of gravity, improving the blood supply to the lungs and brain and giving the legs and heart a rest. Pressure of the abdominal cavity against the diaphragm exercises the diaphragm and heart muscles. Inversions promote better quality of sleep, because they relax the sympathetic nervous system, enabling the relaxation response to kick in.

Twists squeeze, massage and stimulate the organs and muscles; bringing in fresh blood and nutrients; and releasing toxins and wastes. They are also very beneficial in helping to reduce spinal, hip and groin problems.

Forward bends rinse, squeeze and flush the abdominal organs, encouraging proper digestion and elimination, and stretch and tone the organs in the back of the body. They quieten the mind and encourage introspection. The kidneys and adrenals are soothed by forward bends, relieving fatigue and renewing energy.

Backbends squeeze the kidneys and adrenal glands and stretch and tone the organs in the front of the body. The lungs and heart are opened, bringing more breath and circulation throughout the body.

The heart is exercised by the different postures, with many similar benefits as aerobic exercise – with one important exception: through yoga postures, the heart is not stressed as it is in aerobic activities such as running or spinning. The heart receives the actions of the various postures (through toning, stimulating and massaging actions).

In a recent study reported by the American magazine *Yoga Journal,* a group of people who walked for 20 minutes a day three times a week were compared to a group of yoga practitioners who did standing poses for 20 minutes a day, three times a week. Guess who received the greater cardiovascular benefit? The yogis did!

Yoga Benefits for Women

Yoga is fabulous for women of all ages. Many of the poses are terrific for the health of the reproductive organs. It is therapeutic for menstrual, perimenopausal and menopausal symptoms. A relaxing menstruation practice focuses on resting the abdominal area and emphasizes supported seated forward bends, wide-legged poses and basic supported backbends, which help lessen backache, cramp, fatigue and excessive bleeding. Perimenopausal and menopausal women frequently experience mood swings, insomnia, fatigue, hot flushes, redistribution of body fat and irregular bleeding. An appropriate yoga practice can alleviate and reduce many of these symptoms. (See Chapter 21 for the menstruation and perimenopausal/menopausal sequences.)

Yoga Benefits for Men

In general, men have dense, bulky, tight muscles. Yoga postures can go a long way toward loosening and lengthening those knotty muscles. As men approach middle age, many experience prostate problems. Practising a variety of postures, particularly forward bends and poses that open the pelvis and hips, is preventive health for the prostate glands and the lymph glands. (The lymphatic system, which circulates lymph fluid and picks up and eliminates waste throughout the body, greatly benefits from yoga postures and breathing exercises. The lymphatic system does not move on its own. It has to be pumped by the muscles.)

Relieving Chronic Ailments and Reducing Stress

Common chronic ailments – such as arthritis, osteoporosis, obesity, asthma, heart disease, addictions, back problems, knee injuries, arthritis, carpal tunnel syndrome, mild depression, sinus problems and headaches (to name just a few problems!) – can be relieved through regular Hatha Yoga practice.

Yoga for cancer patients emphasizes stress management utilizing awareness, centring and breathing techniques; gentle movement; deep relaxation; and meditation; and it is also used for healing in conjunction with other therapies. These specific yoga techniques help cancer patients to cope with the stress of the disease and with the effects of their treatment such as fatigue, nausea, flu-like symptoms and chemotherapy-induced menopause.

People with multiple sclerosis have found yoga to be extremely beneficial in maintaining muscle, tone, strength and flexibility. Yoga also helps restore a sense of control over their lives and enhances their overall quality of life.

Yoga Helps You Relax

Specific breathing techniques called *pranayama* control the breath and, ultimately, the mind. Pranayama invigorates the entire body-mind system. The respiratory and nervous systems are calmed and strengthened, and all the cells receive the life force and nutrients from the breath. The practice of pranayama, when done correctly, is said to have many curative benefits. The body's vital energy is balanced and replenished. Fatigue is lessened. The mind and the emotions experience calmness and quietness.

Conscious relaxation techniques systematically guide you into a state of deep relaxation. As the noisy chatter of your mind recedes, your body is able to let go and release muscular tension. As your body lets go, the breath rate slows and deepens, so the respiratory system is allowed to rest. Slow, deep breathing encourages relaxation and calmness just as a quick, shallow breath invites anxiety and action.

As the breath rate slows down, the heartbeat responds and also becomes slower. This positively affects the entire circulatory system and rests the heart, allowing it to rejuvenate. The sympathetic nervous system, always ready to gear up for action, gets the message that it is all right to relax, and then the parasympathetic nervous system initiates the relaxation response.

The endocrine glands, responsible for much of your emotional and physical well-being, receive the message to relax. (In this stress-driven society, the adrenal glands in particular become overused and depleted.)

This deep relaxation goes to the very core of decreasing fatigue and unravelling you from the inside out like a knotted ball of twine. You emerge from this experience full of energy, as if you've just returned from a mini-break from your stressful life.

Inner Fulfilment

Meditation, a part of yoga, is a powerful tool for reducing tension and stress and for bringing you back in touch with your true self and your inner reality. In meditation, you sit and watch the workings of the mind as a dispassionate observer. Through meditation you observe the fluctuations of the mind and realize the preciousness of the present moment. The events of the past and the future loosen their grip on you, and everyday concerns take a back seat as you focus on yourself. The frenetic pace of life slows down and becomes manageable, even peaceful. What seemed so earth-shattering just minutes ago is now put into perspective. You become aware of thought patterns and the vacillation of human emotions.

In meditation, the innate intelligence and awareness of the individual are awakened. New thoughts and ways of being emerge. (The body is also learning new patterns of movement through yoga postures.) What people perceive as the mind permeates every cell in the body, and does not simply reside in the head. Through meditation, the mind-body system is unified and the individual is one step closer to the realization of oneness and unity with all other beings, known as *unitive consciousness.*

This is a material world, where external achievement and the accumulation of wealth in the form of money and possessions are the main measure of success. Greed and excessive consumption are rampant. Computers and television passively entertain and isolate. Immediate gratification appears to be at our fingertips. Unfortunately, this route leads to alienation from the real, internal self, with the resulting feelings of emptiness and apathy. The practice of Hatha Yoga can help fill this void by offering a path to inner fulfilment and spirituality.

Disorders such as bulimia and anorexia, overeating, over-exercising and abuse of credit cards, alcohol and drugs are desperate, unconscious and unsuccessful attempts to fill the void caused by this unbalanced lifestyle. External rewards are only temporary fixes that do not feed the need for connection to yourself and the common good.

Self-Esteem and Body Image

Hatha Yoga helps develop positive self-esteem, body image and a more comfortable and realistic view of yourself. This is sorely needed in a world in which you are incessantly bombarded by media images of thin, beautiful, air-brushed models and celebrities (truly the impossible dream for most ordinary people).

The practice of yoga creates physical, mental and emotional confidence and stability. The body becomes stronger and more agile. The mind begins to listen to the needs of the body and cultivates a mind-body relationship. Self-esteem and confidence grow. The inner voice is awakened. Understanding of your emotions deepens. The need to stuff emotions out of consciousness through overeating, or to be in control by starving the body, diminishes. As you listen internally, you begin responding to appropriate internal cues and eating nutritious foods when you're hungry, contributing positively to your overall health.

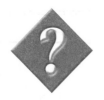

Can yoga help me lose weight?
Yes, but probably not in the way you'd expect. It's not the poses themselves that help you lose weight. It's the attitude you develop from the practice of yoga. Yoga allows you to relax, enjoy and begin to eat in a controlled way that is natural and self-regulating.

Improved Posture

Hatha Yoga improves your posture in daily life. Yoga students frequently comment that, as a result of doing yoga, they become increasingly aware of their posture and correct it during daily activities outside class. Better physical alignment and posture is visually appealing and also says a lot about a person, but the effects go much deeper.

A person with rounded shoulders will have trouble breathing fully because the chest is collapsed. This is also the posture of a depressed, overwhelmed person, who may have neck discomfort because the neck's natural curve has changed as a result of poor postural habits. Someone with a *sway back* (an exaggerated lower back curve) may experience low back pain as a result of a forward tilting pelvis and shortened, tight lower-back muscles, and possibly suffer from compression in the lower back.

When the body is in good alignment, the bones stack up properly from the feet up. If the *femur* (thigh) bones insert properly into the pelvis, the hips will be level with each other and create a balanced sacrum, crucial to the alignment and health of the spine. The *sacrum* is the fulcrum upon which the spine rests.

Many people experience chronic back pain as a result of sacrum dysfunction. A balanced spine arising out of the pelvis will ensure that the torso is well supported and free to bend in all directions. When the bones insert properly into the joints, the muscles can fall into place and work in a balanced, coordinated manner, and the organs will have enough space to function optimally.

A physically aligned body promotes mental, emotional and spiritual alignment and clarity. For example, how many times have you had a headache, neck ache or backache and found it impossible to concentrate or think? Didn't you become irritable and short-tempered? Yoga helps prevent that.

Increased Bone Density

A recent study in the United States, conducted by Professor Steven A. Hawkins and faculty yoga teacher Bee Beckman of the Department of Kinesiology and Physical Education at California State University, worked with 18 women from 18 to 65 years of age who had no former yoga experience. Half the group participated in two yoga classes a week and also practised by themselves three times a week. Some of the required poses practiced were triangle, half moon, extended side angle,and warriors I and II. The women in the control group had to continue their normal level of activity throughout the study.

Bone density scans were done at the beginning of the study and then six months later. After six months, in the yoga group bone density of the spine increased significantly, while those in the control group had no change in their bone density levels. More studies with larger population groups are needed to get a clearer picture, but it is evident that weight-bearing yoga postures (arm balances, inversions and standing poses) maintain bone density, increase bone density, and help prevent osteoporosis and fragile bones.

Stress, not surprisingly, affects bone density adversely. Overdoing aerobic activity leads to decreased body fat and increases the likelihood of osteoporosis. Living a stressful lifestyle full of adrenaline rushes depletes calcium and imbalances hormonal activity. A consistent yoga practice, which includes weight-bearing and restorative postures, relaxation and meditation, helps lessen the effects of stress and restores balance.

Emotional Balance

Hatha Yoga has a profound impact upon the emotions. Forward bends are introverted postures and thus have a quieting effect, reducing agitation and anxiety. Backbends are extroverted postures that are exhilarating, help open the body and release held emotions such as sadness and grief. Inversions turn your world upside down literally, and allow you to change your perspective on life – they are mood elevators. Twists are cleansing. Specific breathing exercises can be done to calm or energize the individual. Relaxation and meditation practices are also extremely useful, depending upon the situation.

Of course, yoga is *not* a substitute for mental therapy. Mental health professionals should be utilized when necessary. The combination of yoga and psychotherapy can be a very powerful accelerator to personal healing and growth as the mind and the body are jointly explored and united.

Improved Sex Life

The physical yoga postures stimulate and strengthen the body and improve circulation. The pelvic organs and the muscles supporting them, particularly the perineal muscles (located between the anus and the genitals) and the pelvic floor are toned, oxygenated and flushed with fresh blood and nutrients. This can contribute to greater sensitivity and responsiveness during intercourse.

Tight areas, such as shoulders, hips, hamstrings, groins and lower backs, loosen and become more flexible. Greater flexibility allows for a greater variety of sexual positions and ease of movement.

Body image and self-esteem frequently improve as a result of doing yoga, and this can only enhance and improve your sex life. Very often people are inhibited and self-conscious of how their bodies look and how their partners might react. People tend to think that their physical appearance and performance are being judged during sex. This attitude can be a total turn-off for both you and your partner, because it does not allow you to be playful and focus on the fun you might have together if you weren't so concerned with your external appearance. Being comfortable in your own skin makes a big difference in how you interact on an intimate level – and yoga can help.

The physical postures, breathing exercises, deep relaxation and meditation help decrease fatigue and stress and promote relaxation. Less stress and fatigue translate into less irritability, more patience, and greater energy and emotional availability. A greater ability to relax helps to decrease inhibitions and increase sexual spontaneity and fun in bed.

Yoga focuses the mind. A wandering mind during sex does not allow you to be fully present and intimate with your partner. It might make for a great fantasy life, but not for loving the one you're with!

CHAPTER 3

The History of Yoga

Yoga originated over 5,000 years ago as an oral tradition passed on from teacher to student. In India in the 1920s, archaeologists discovered the Indus civilization, the largest civilization in antiquity, which helped them to date the beginnings of yoga. Some of the ruins contained yogic figures engraved on soapstone seals.

The Four Yogic Periods

It is now believed that Yoga developed within a mature civilization that flourished for many years, until tectonic changes in the earth dried up the famous Sarasvati River, immortalized in the oldest known Indo-European text, the *Rig-Veda*. This famous text is written in Sanskrit, the ancient language of most yoga scriptures. The history of yoga can be grouped into four sequential yogic time periods: Vedic, Preclassical, Classical and Postclassical.

Today, a wide diversity of people from all walks of life try yoga for a variety of reasons. There are many wonderful yoga teachers and styles of yoga for anyone. The classical styles of yoga remain, but new styles are constantly evolving.

Vedic Yoga

Vedic Yoga, also know as *Archaic Yoga,* was practised during the time of the *Rig-Veda* teachings. *Veda* means 'knowledge' and *rig* means 'praise'. The *Rig-Veda* is a compilation of hymns that praise a higher power.

Vedic Yoga centred on ritualistic ceremonies – some involving sacrifice – as a means to join matter with spirit. These ritualistic activities, which are the roots of yoga, required the practitioner to focus inward to transcend the limitations of the mind. Some Vedic Yogi masters called *seers* or *rishis* experienced 'visions', which transcended reality.

Preclassical Yoga

Preclassical Yoga is a broad time period spanning 2,000 years up to the 2nd century AD. The earliest part of this time period was strongly influenced by ritualistic Vedic culture. The *Upanishads,* a text of sacred revelations exploring the hidden teachings and the interconnectedness of all things in the universe, was written during this time. The *Bhagavad-Gita,* composed around 500BC, teaches that one must lead an active life full of benign actions, opposing evil and going beyond the control of the ego.

Many schools during this time taught various techniques for reaching deep levels of meditation, with the goal of transcending the mind-body system toward the true, limitless self.

Classical Yoga

Classical Yoga describes the eight-limbed path of yoga, also known as *Raja Yoga,* the royal path. This is the yoga Patanjali writes about in the classical treatise, the *Yoga Sutra (sutra* meaning 'thread'), a text of 195 aphorisms elucidating the philosophy of Yoga. The *Yoga Sutra* was meant to be recited and memorized as a means of internalizing its wisdom.

It is thought that the *Yoga Sutra* was written in the 2nd century AD. Not much is known about its author, Patanjali. He is described as a grammarian, physician and philosopher. Over the years, there have been countless explanations and translations of the *Yoga Sutra.*

Postclassical Yoga

Postclassical Yoga includes the many different schools of yoga that arose after Patanjali's time. At this time, yoga adepts began exploring the body as a vehicle used to attain liberation and merge with the spirit. Before this time, the body was thought of only as a container of the spirit, with the goal of energizing and revitalizing the body to prolong its life. The body was now seen as a temple that housed the spirit and, therefore, should be well taken care of and kept clean and healthy. This mode of thought led to the creation of Hatha Yoga and to the different schools of Tantra Yoga.

Yoga's Recent History

The modern yoga time period could be said to being in the West with the Parliament of Religions in Chicago during 1893, where Swami (meaning 'master') Vivekenanda inspired the American people. After this event, he travelled widely and wrote several books, drawing many students to yoga. Vivekenanda's widespread influence stimulated tremendous interest in Eastern philosophies, which continues to this day.

Paramahansa Yogananada, author of *Autobiography of a Yogi,* was another popular Yoga teacher. He went to the United States in 1920, and established the Self-Realization Fellowship, which has grown to have a worldwide following.

From the early 1930s until he died in 1986, Jiddu Krishnamurti inspired thousands of Westerners, who were seeking knowledge, spirituality, and truth, through his writings and talks. Greta Garbo, Charlie Chaplin and Aldous Huxley were among his close friends, and Bernard Shaw described Krishnamurti as 'the most beautiful human being' he ever saw.

Hatha Yoga was introduced into America by Russian-born Indra Devi, the 'first lady of yoga', who opened her first yoga studio in 1947. Indra was the first non-Indian and first woman to learn the yogic teachings and bring them to the West. She taught many celebrities at her studio and trained hundreds of teachers. Indra lived and opened studios in several other countries, and lived and taught in Argentina until her death in 2002, aged 102.

In 1947, Theos Bernard, who studied yoga in India, published *Hatha Yoga: The Report of a Personal Experience.* This account became a reference book for yoga throughout the 1950s.

Selvarajan Yesudian was a well-known yoga teacher in the 1950s, whose book *Sport and Yoga* sold 50,000 copies and was translated into 15 languages. Today, many professional athletes continue to use yoga to help prevent injuries, focus their minds and improve their overall athletic performance.

Richard Hittelman hosted yoga on television in 1961, and this was particularly popular in the United Kingdom. This pioneering effort, as well as the best-selling book he wrote, called *The Twenty-Eight-Day Yoga Plan,* which sold millions of copies, greatly influenced thoughts about yoga around the world. Although he was spiritually based in yoga, Richard taught a type of yoga that emphasized health benefits.

In the mid-1960s, the Beatles became involved briefly with Maharishi Mahesh Yogi and his form of Transcendental Meditation (TM). Their relationship with the Maharishi sparked tremendous interest in yoga. Thousands of people all over the world practiced TM, and many more were introduced to meditation as a result. Medical research involving meditation began at this time.

In 1967, B.K.S. Iyengar wrote the classic yoga text for serious yoga students, *Light on Yoga*. B.K.S. Iyengar's emphasis on anatomical precision and correct alignment in postures, as well as the use of equipment for therapeutic and restorative purposes, and for obtaining the best pose possible, had a massive impact on the way yoga was taught all over the world.

In the 1960s and 1970s, disciples of the Himalayan master, Swami Sivananada, opened schools in Europe and America. The disciples are:

· Swami Vishnudevananda, author of the popular book *The Complete Illustrated Book of Yoga*.
· Swami Satchitananada, who introduced chanting and yoga at Woodstock.
· Swami Sivananda Radha, a female swami who studied the connection between yoga and psychology.
· Swami Satyananda and Swami Chidananda, of the Sivananda Ashram in Rishkesh, India.

Other important Indian Yoga masters of this time include:

· Sri Aurobindo, the founder of Integral Yoga
· Ramana Maharshi, master of Jnana-Yoga
· Papa Ramdas, of Mantra-Yoga
· Swami Nityananda, of Siddha-Yoga
· Swami Mutkananda, a student of Swami Nityananda, who familiarized Westerners with Siddha Yoga

Sri Krishnamacharya

The great Hatha Yoga master Sri Krishnamacharya was a scholar of yoga, Sanskrit, Ayurveda and the healing arts. He utilized yoga as therapy, describing it as 'healing without surgery'. There is no Hatha Yoga that hasn't been influenced by Krishnamacharya, through the lineage of teachers he trained. Krishnamacharya was descended from a revered 9th-century yogi named Nathamuni. His father began teaching him the *Yoga Sutras* at the tender age of five. When Krishnamacharya was 16, he made a pilgrimage to the shrine of Nathamuni. There Krishnamacharya had a vision of Nathamuni, who taught him verses from the *Yogarahasya (The Essence of Yoga),* which Krishnamacharya memorized and later transcribed. This ancient text provided the basis of Krishnamacharya's teachings.

Following this experience, Krishnamacharya continued his education, receiving degrees in philology, logic, divinity and music. He continued his study of yoga on his own, but yearned for guidance and instruction. A teacher suggested that he seek out a yoga master by the name of Sri Ramamohan Brahmachari. (At this time, there were very few Hatha Yoga masters alive.) Krishnamacharya lived with Brahmachari and his family for seven years, memorizing the *Yoga Sutra,* learning asanas, pranayama and the therapeutics of yoga. His teacher never asked Krishnamacharya for payment. Instead, Brahmacharya instructed Krishnamacharya to return to the world, marry and teach yoga.

Krishnamacharya began teaching and married by arrangement. For many years, he and his wife lived in poverty, because teaching yoga was not profitable. When he wasn't teaching, Krishnamacharya would travel and give demonstrations and lectures to help popularize yoga. He would demonstrate supra-normal abilities, such as stopping his pulse, stopping cars with his bare hands and lifting heavy things with his teeth. Finally, he was well compensated and could teach yoga full time. The Maharaja of Mysore helped Krishnamacharya publicize yoga for the next 20 years. After this time, Krishnamacharya was offered the use of the palace's gymnastics hall as his yoga school.

Krishnamacharya developed what is now called Ashtanga Vinyasa Yoga, a style that emphasizes flowing postures coordinated with the breath, and divided into three series: primary, intermediate and advanced. Pattabhi Jois, one of Krishnamacharya's students, took this style of practice and popularized it (it is known as *Ashtanga Yoga*).

After much persistence, Indra Devi became Krishnamacharya's first Western female student. He taught her yoga instruction, diet and pranayama. At this time in his life, Krishnamacharya was teaching a gentler type of yoga, focusing on the sequencing of postures.

B.K.S. Iyengar received instruction from Krishnamacharya for only a short period of time. However, he was deeply influenced by Krishnamacharya. Indeed, both greatly emphasized the therapeutic benefits of yoga. Afterwards, Iyengar would practice and explore the poses using his own body. He utilized a wide variety of natural props, such as steamrollers for back bends and heavy cobblestones to force his legs into Baddha Konasana (cobbler pose). His wife, Ramamani, worked with him in his experimentation with the asanas. Iyengar is known worldwide as both a teacher and a healer.

Iyengar developed a style of yoga that was intensely introspective and focused on detailed anatomical articulation of the asanas, the development of specific therapeutic yoga sequences, and his rigorous, many-levelled teacher training system. His Hatha Yoga style has deeply affected every type of Hatha Yoga. He certainly has had an amazing impact upon the West's fascination with and practice of yoga.

Krishnamacharya's last major student and disciple was his own son. T.K.V. Desikachar, trained as an engineer, originally felt no urge to teach yoga, and when he did, his father tried to dissuade him. Thus began 28 years of study, with Krishnamacharya tutoring his son. During this time, Krishnamacharya was refining his approach, now called *Viniyoga*. This style emphasized an individualized focus, tailoring practice to the therapeutic needs of the student. Practice was now divided into three life stages: youth, middle and old age. As students progressed, the spiritual aspect of practice was stressed, while respecting an individual's cultural background.

Not sure that yoga really changes your body? In 1970, researchers at the Menninger Foundation were astonished when Swami Rama was able to control the functions of his autonomic nervous system, including his heartbeat, pulse and skin temperature.

Krishnamacharya's legacy is that he was able to respect the past teachings of yoga and adapt them to meet modern needs. Through this willingness to experiment and refine, he and his teachers have brought yoga to millions around the world. He died in 1998, and today his son Desikachar, carries on his legacy, teaching at the Krishnamacharya Yoga Mandiram, in Chennai, India, and teaching Viniyoga to teachers and students all over the world.

CHAPTER 4
Yoga Philosophy

The philosophy of yoga is like a living, breathing organism passed on from teacher to student for many generations over the last 5,000 years. Patanjali, the sage, is credited with compiling and codifying the basic tenets of yoga philosophy into a coherent unified text called the *Yoga Sutra*.

The Six Branches of Yoga

Over the ages yoga has been likened to a tree with roots, a trunk, branches, blossoms and fruits. Yoga has six different branches: Raja, Karma, Bhakti, Jnana, Tantra and Hatha. Each branch has distinctive approaches that make it more or less appropriate for an individual, depending upon his or her personality and learning style. Each path leads to transformational growth and self-actualization. An individual may be involved in one or more paths; they are not mutually exclusive.

Raja Yoga

Raja means 'royal'. Its focus is meditation and contemplation. Many, but not all, practitioners of Raja Yoga live contemplative lives in spiritual communities or religious orders. Raja Yoga is based upon the eight limbs of yoga as discussed in the *Yoga Sutra* (see page 31).

Karma Yoga

Karma Yoga is the path of service. Everyone who is living is on the path of Karma Yoga. Your life is a consequence of your past actions. Therefore, your decisions in life can be consciously chosen to create a future that is free from selfishness and negativity. You are prasticing Karma Yoga whenever you perform a selfless service. Mother Teresa is a good example of someone who provided this kind of selfless service throughout her life.

Bhakti Yoga

Bhakti Yoga is the path of the heart and devotion. A practitioner on this path sees the Divine in everyone and in everything and devotes his life to cultivating acceptance, love and tolerance for all.

Jnana Yoga

Jnana Yoga is the path of wisdom and knowledge. It is the yoga of the mind. Individuals who live life through their intellect will be attracted to this path. Scholars who seriously study the yogic scriptures and texts are Jnana Yogis.

Hatha Yoga

Hatha Yoga is the path of physical yoga. The physical postures, breathing techniques, deep relaxation and meditation comprise Hatha Yoga. Hatha Yoga is the focus of this book.

Tantra Yoga

Tantra Yoga is the path of ritual. It is the most misunderstood path. Part of the tantric path includes rituals for consecrated (or sacred) sexuality. Unfortunately, it is this aspect of Tantric Yoga that has been publicized and blown out of proportion by the media to seem more sexual than it really is. The practice of Tantric Yoga utilizes rituals to reverentially experience the sacred in *everything* we do, not just in sex. It is the most esoteric of all the yogas and attracts those who enjoy ceremony, celebration and ritual.

The Yoga Sutra

According to one of the yoga sutras, yoga is the ability to direct the mind without distraction or interruption. The goal is to reach the state of yoga called *samadhi,* where the mind is crystal-clear and free from impressions of the past or thoughts of the future. Patanjali's *Yoga Sutra* places importance upon how we perceive things and explains why we are always getting into trouble in life. It is our perceptions that colour our view of reality and prevent us from clearly seeing the truth. If we cannot see a situation with clarity, we are unable to act accurately.

Patanjali explains that there are several factors that interfere with our ability to see clearly and accurately. They are comprehension, misapprehension, imagination, memory, deep sleep and memory. Each of these can be beneficial when appropriate and in balance with our needs; otherwise, they can cause problems. For example, our mind fills with misapprehension and fear. We rely too much on our imagination and memory, rather than seeing the simple truth right before our eyes. We may spend too much of our time sleeping.

When you see something correctly, without interference, you feel a deep feeling of calmness and peace. Tension dissolves. Instability and agitation decrease. Over time, you experience longer periods of clarity of thought and emotional stability. Your attitude shifts from negative thoughts and fear to positive thoughts and freedom. You are able to maintain the state of yoga for longer periods of time. Yoga then becomes the practice of examining your habitual attitudes, motives and actions. Yoga is truly a science of the mind.

How to Achieve the State of Yoga

In the *Yoga Sutra,* there are three ways to successfully achieve this state of yoga. The first is through *tapas,* which means 'to heat or cleanse'. *Tapas* in the *Yoga Sutra* refers to the practice of physical postures and breathing exercises. These help release blocks and impurities from the mind and the body in addition to providing many benefits. *Tapas* also refers to a burning desire toward wholeness, self-knowledge and self-integration.

A second way to reach the state of yoga is through self-study or *svadhyaya.* Through *svadhyaya,* we examine and rediscover our true selves. The reading of yoga scriptures and texts helps with this self-study. We also observe our thoughts, actions and reactions when doing yoga as well as in daily life.

The third approach is *isvarapranidhana,* translated as 'love of God'. There is an element of surrender and devotion in *isvarapranidhana,* which occurs during the process of committing oneself to the path of yoga. This surrender happens again and again as your practice and growth through yoga deepens. *Isvarapranidhana* also means a certain quality of action. Practising postures and breathing techniques along with self-study is not enough to reach the state of yoga. You must continue living your daily life, working and living with others in a way that is positive and loving. All three approaches constitute the yoga of attentive action known as *Kriya Yoga.*

tips

These three approaches are tiers that occur throughout each stage or limb of yoga. First, there must be *sadhana,* or practice. *Sadhana is* essential for the three tiers to occur. After practice is established, the foundation has been set for *tapas, svadhyaya* and *isvarapranidhana.*

The Eight Limbs of Yoga

Patanjali uses the word *limb* to describe the different aspects of yogic practice that, when taken together, make up one body of Yoga. The purpose of this eight-fold path is as a practical guide to self-development that helps to bring the mind, body and spirit into harmony. Each limb can grow at the same or different time. They develop together spontaneously in a process that is developmental, harmonious and organic. The limbs are:

- **Yamas:** Your attitudes toward others outside yourself or universal laws
- **Niyamas:** Your attitude about yourself or your personal observances
- **Asanas:** Physical postures
- **Pranayama:** Regulation and control of the breath
- **Pratyahara:** Withdrawal of the senses
- **Dharana:** Concentration
- **Dhyana:** Meditation
- **Samadhi:** Self-realization or enlightenment

These limbs are not sequential rungs of a ladder that must be climbed from bottom to top. You can begin with any limb and experience the other limbs at any time. All the limbs lead to the same destination, *samadhi.*

What distracts us from the path of yoga?
According to Patanjali, illness, mental stagnation, doubts, lack of foresight, overindulgence, illusion about one's true state of mind, lack of perseverance and regression are the nine symptoms that distract us from the path of yoga.

Yamas: Universal Laws

The yamas are the roots of the tree of yoga. They provide the foundation for the practice of yoga.

Ahimsa

The first yama is *ahimsa*. Ahimsa means 'non-harming, non-violence'. But it is much more than that. To observe ahimsa is to practise kindness, friendliness and thoughtfulness toward others and yourself. Ahimsa includes observing whether your thoughts and actions are leading to your personal growth and the welfare of all beings. It is about living life peacefully without fear. Some may interpret ahimsa as not eating meat, wearing animal skins and so on, but this is a matter of personal preference and decision.

Not harming yourself and others could also mean providing food and shelter for your family and physically defending yourself from danger. Each circumstance must be acted upon independently and with flexibility of thought and awareness, while keeping the principles of ahimsa in your mind.

Ahimsa isn't just about your treatment of others. You would be practicing ahimsa when doing yoga postures in a way that did not cause injury or harm to *yourself*. Honouring the body's needs at each moment in time, listening and responding appropriately, is practising ahimsa. This means not pushing beyond your range of comfort.

Satya

The next yama is *satya* or 'truthfulness'. Satya means 'to speak the truth'. However, it is not always possible to speak the truth, because the truth may be harmful to another person. It is important to think before you speak and consider the consequences of your words. If speaking the truth would be destructive to another person, it might be better to say nothing rather than tell a lie. Gossiping can be considered harmful to the person receiving it. In this way satya would be in alignment with the principle of ahimsa (non-harming).

Satya can be seen as living a truthful life that is in alignment with your own needs and abilities. Someone who is unhappy with his job, his marriage or his relationship is not living his life in accordance with satya.

Asteya

Asteya is the third yama. It means 'non-stealing' or 'not taking what does not belong to us'. Asteya refers to non-stealing of material things, as well as of another's ideas. If someone confides in you, it would be appropriate to keep the confidence rather than break it by telling someone else the confidential information.

Asteya encompasses misappropriation, mismanagement and mistrust, and involves the misuse of power. Using power in a way that is self-serving, rather than for the good of others, would not be practising asteya. Machiavelli's 'the end justifies the means' is not in accordance with asteya.

Bramacharya

The fourth yama is *bramacharya,* which means 'to move towards the essential truth'. Bramacharya has commonly been seen as self-control, abstinence or moderation, especially regarding sexual activity. Sexual energy is more than the act of sexual union and those activities related to it. It is the creative power of each person.

Celibacy has been thought of as bramacharya, but it is really moderation of the senses and desires that is most important. Bramacharya is about conserving your creative energies so they are not dissipated.

The *Yoga Sutra* cautions that giving into the ego's excessive desires can lead us far off the path of yoga. We are told that it is responsible behaviour that moves us to our truth. Remember the second statement of the oracles found at Delphi: 'Nothing in excess'. This also applies to our yoga practice. Life should be full of health, balance and harmony.

Aparigraha

Aparigraha, the last yama, means 'to take only what is necessary and not to take advantage of someone or of a situation'. It implies non-hoarding, and faith and trust in what life has to offer each one of us. We are asked to take what we have earned fairly, not to ask for an excessive amount for our efforts. It is about learning to live a simple, contented life, satisfied with what you have, and believing that you will be given all that you need. Aparigraha refers to using one's power correctly and appropriately, not exploiting someone else. It is all about correct use of power.

The student-teacher relationship in yoga must be one of aparigraha. It is an intimate relationship in which the teacher is guiding the student in self-evolution and discovery. The teacher must treat each student fairly, with compassion and respect. The student has put his trust in the teacher and it must not be abused or taken advantage of. Although a student relies upon his teacher's knowledge and expertise, this should not translate into an unhealthy dependence or servitude. The teacher is to be respected, but it is important to remember that we are all students of life, with no one superior to the other.

Niyamas: Personal Observances

The second limb of yoga is the *niyamas*. They are personal observances toward ourselves. Niyamas are the trunk of the tree of Yoga. They control the senses of perception, the eyes, ears, nose, mouth, tongue and skin.

Sauca

The first niyama is *sauca,* or 'cleanliness'. Sauca implies both inner and outer cleanliness, of our internal and external environments. Inner cleanliness is of utmost importance for preserving the healthy functioning of every body system. The physical postures, breathing techniques and yogic cleansing practices irrigate and detoxify the physical body.

The mind must also be kept clean. Holding onto old thoughts and ways of perceiving can clutter the mind, making it difficult to think clearly. Spring cleaning of the mind is needed.

Outer cleanliness of our environment provides the proper home for an uncluttered mind. Practicing yoga postures, yogic cleansing techniques, and breathing exercises are essential for maintaining inner sauca and eliminating what is no longer necessary.

Yogic cleansing techniques, called *shatkriya*, were developed to prepare the student for yoga and were taught only by an advanced teacher. There are techniques beneficial for excess mucus, excess fat or an imbalance in the body *doshas (vatta, pitta* and *kapha)* when asana or pranayama do not solve the problem. They are covered in the following sections. **Note that these techniques should be done under the supervision of a qualified yoga professional.**

Neti: The Nasal Wash

The sinus cavity and nasal passages are cleansed with a warm saline solution (1/2 teaspoon of salt in lukewarm water) best done with a *neti pot*, a small, ceramic vessel that looks like Aladdin's lamp with a shorter spout. Turning the head to one side at a sink, lukewarm water is poured into one nostril and flows out the other nostril while breathing through the mouth. Then the other side is similarly irrigated. The procedure can also be done nostril-to-mouth and mouth-to-nostril, and is effective in relieving sinus headaches and allergies. It also enhances ease of breathing for pranayama. Neti cleansing, called *sutra neti*, can also be performed with a string or catheter under guided supervision.

Dhauti: Gastrointestinal Cleansing

Gastrointestinal cleansing, known as *dhauti*, consists of upper and lower washing of the internal body with a lukewarm saline solution. 4.5–9l (1–2gal) of salt water are swallowed for the upper body wash. Then the salt water is regurgitated, resulting in a cleansing of the entire mucus lining of the upper respiratory tract. This procedure is recommended for people with chronic respiratory conditions.

The lower body wash of one to two gallons of lukewarm salt water is also swallowed, but is allowed to be excreted through the body's excretory system, aided by particular yogic movements to stimulate the digestive process and cleanse the lower digestive tract. Both techniques should be done seasonally to keep the internal body clean and healthy.

Basti: Cleansing of the Bowel

Cleansing of the bowel, called *basti,* is performed for the health of the bowels. *Jala basti* is a yogic enema, again, best done under the supervision of a knowledgeable yoga professional.

Trataka: Gazing

Gazing, or *trataka,* encompasses a number of practices that involve focusing upon an object, such as a candle, for an extended length of time. This practice results in an increased ability to focus one's attention and purify the mind. Note that this should not be attempted by persons suffering from epilepsy or depression, or with a mental disorder.

Nauli: Abdominal Churning

Abdominal churning, known as *nauli,* involves utilizing a pumping and churning action of the abdominal muscles and organs to cleanse, strengthen and energize the abdominal area. The practitioner must be familiar and practiced in this and similar techniques.

Kapalbhati: Skull Shining Breath

Skull shining breath, or *kapalbhati,* is a vigorous breathing exercise. It cleanses the abdominal organs, lungs, nasal sinuses and passages, and strengthens the heart and nervous system.

Samtosha

Samtosha, the second niyama, means being modest, humble and content with who we are and with what we have in this life. *Samtosha* also means to accept what happens in life, rather than rigidly pursuing a specific goal or an expectation of how things are supposed to be. Samtosha is all about enjoying the process and the journey through life, taking time to smell the roses. This includes practising yoga in a process-oriented way, not as a goal-directed activity.

Tapas

The next niyama is *tapas,* discussed earlier in this chapter. The burning or cleansing action of tapas refers to keeping the body in good condition. Through tapas, the body rids itself of impurities of the mind (thought) and the body. This includes carefully paying attention to what you put into your body in the way of food, medications, what you read, what you view on television or in films, and what you think.

Eating only when you are hungry, maintaining good posture and patterns of movement, and establishing smooth, regular breathing all constitute the practice of tapas. Tapas also refers to the burning away of thoughts, desires and wants that do not truly serve the individual.

Purification occurs on the physical, emotional, mental and spiritual planes. It does not include self-denial and should not cause suffering. The yogic science of diet acknowledges food as an important source of *prana,* or vital energy. You receive energy from the food you eat and the air you breathe. Your body is your only vehicle in this lifetime, and you have to take good care of it so it will last a long time. As a human being who is becoming more self-aware and knowledgeable of your own needs, conscious eating is a way to bring yoga practice into your daily life. The yoga of conscious eating emphasizes eating the right kind of food, which balances your nutritional needs and is chosen by inner cues regarding what the body naturally craves, not by habitual desires. Whole foods, fruits, vegetables and grains, and fish and meat that are minimally processed or exposed to antibiotics and hormones are good food choices that contain the most prana. Highly processed snack foods and canned items do not provide the body with adequate nourishment. They may temporarily appease your taste buds, but your inner chemistry is brought out of balance by these empty foods.

Eating the correct quantity of food is another important component of the yoga of conscious eating. Most of us live in a society in which there is an abundance of food available. We frequently eat automatically, habitually and socially. Overeating is easy, constantly tempted by television commercials and infinite choices down seemingly endless supermarket aisles. Often we watch television, read or eat quickly. We may also eat when emotionally upset. We eat for emotional reasons, either looking for something sweet in our lives or using food to put down unpleasant emotions out of our consciousness. As a result, our senses are dulled and we are not aware of how much we are eating or what it tastes like. We are encouraged to be excessive and hoard food, but remember, moderation, or *bramacharya,* is the key.

Don't forget how to listen to your inner cues of hunger and feeling full. Frequent snacking does not allow efficient digestion and elimination of food and waste products. The digestive system needs to do its job and then rest.

A final component of the yoga of conscious eating is the idea that food is sustenance. The development of effective eating habits, such as eating only when hungry, eating slowly, chewing completely before swallowing, and filling the stomach two-thirds full (some say that at each meal we should eat the volume of our fist, since it is the size of our stomach), will enable the digestive system to break down, assimilate and eliminate food as efficiently and smoothly as possible. When you eat slowly, the internal feeling of satiation is felt at the appropriate time and you are able to control overeating. The digestive fire is strongest during midday. It is during this time that the largest meal of the day should be consumed.

To help bring your eating habits into conscious awareness, ask yourself the followkng questions:

- Am I hungry now?
- Am I eating just because it's time to eat a meal?
- Am I enjoying this meal?
- Am I eating in front of the television, or reading something, instead of focusing solely on my meal?

· Am I responding to other people's needs or giving into society's pressures by eating these foods, or eating at this time?
· What emotions do I associate with this food choice?
· Am I eating out of frustration or tension, and if so, what do I eat when I feel this way?
· When I feel relaxed what do I feel like eating?
· Is there another activity besides eating that I could do to satisfy my needs at this time?

Remember that conscious eating is a way of developing greater sensitivity to your needs. It reflects how you are in relationship to yourself. Can you translate the caring and compassion that you show others to yourself?

The principles of conscious eating are:

- Eat in moderation.
- Eat only when hungry.
- Eat in a relaxed and quiet environment.
- Drink liquids that are warm or at room temperature.
- Keep a variety of nutritious, wholesome foods in the house, such as fresh fruits, vegetables and whole grains.
- Do not eat processed snack foods.
- Eat fewer sugary and salty foods.
- Make dietary changes gradually.

Svadhyaya

Svadhyaya is the fourth niyama, which is described as self-study, self-inquiry or self-examination. Any learning that allows you to get to know yourself more completely is svadhyaya. This includes study of spiritual texts, chanting, prayers and spending time with nature.

In yoga, you become very intimate with yourself, discovering all kinds of things you may not have been aware of previously. It is the awakening of the innate intelligence within and the expansion of total awareness with clarity. The *Yoga Sutra* states that as you grow in self-knowledge, you will be able to deepen your self-knowledge, your connection to the Divine (a higher power) and your interconnectedness with all things.

Isvarapranidhana

The last niyama is *isvarapranidhana,* which means 'to lay all your actions at the feet of God'. As we grow in awareness and experience the unpredictability of life, we realize that we are really not in control. Isvarapranidhana addresses this and encourages you to surrender your life and false sense of control to whatever you connect to that gives you a sense of wholeness and sacredness, whether that be in the form of God or nature. Offering prayer is a way of acknowledging the role of isvarapranidhana in our lives.

Asana: Physical Postures

The third limb of yoga is *asana.* Asanas are the branches of the tree of yoga, which bring the physical and physiological functions of the body into harmony with the psychological aspect. These are the physical postures that relax, rejuvenate, strengthen and energize the body. There are more than 80 postures (and many variations) designed for this purpose.

Many of the asanas are named after animals and plant life (for example, dog pose, cobra pose, tree pose and crow pose). Other postures are named after sages, gods and stars. The poses represent the principles of evolution, with the body taking the various forms and evolving. One theory explaining the development of the asanas is that the yogis lived close to nature, studying their fellow creatures and the earth and sky surrounding them. The yogis were particularly fascinated with the way sick animals moved their bodies in an effort to feel better, and the asanas reflect these successful adaptations of intrinsic animal movement and intelligence. Another theory says that the yogis, who sat for hours and meditated, spontaneously went into asanas as the kundalini energy rose up the spine, and that this is how the asanas were organically created.

In the *Yoga Sutra* it is said that the asanas are to be done with steadiness, alertness and comfort, achieving a balance between ease and effort. The asanas are consciously linked with the flow of the breath, with each movement inspired by the breath. The practice of the asana is inner-directed, with the practitioner being the observer *and* the observed, paying attention to himself and his actions.

As you practise the asanas and learn from yoga instructors, you may hear the word *chakra* used. Chakra is Sanskrit for 'wheel of light'. The chakras are energy centres, likened to spinning vortexes, which conduct electromagnetic energy. There are seven chakra bodies: the physical body, the mental body, the emotional body, the intellectual body, the astral body, the aetheric body and the ketheric body. The astral body, located at the heart centre, is the bridge between matter and spirit. It is the integration of these seven bodies that occurs in yoga.

There are seven main chakras or energy centres in the subtle body, located along the spine, and 122 smaller chakras throughout the body. The seven chakras correspond to the major glands in the physical body, to major nerve plexuses and to specific colours, depending upon the frequency that each chakra spins.

Each chakra in the subtle body is recognized as a concentrated point of life force, relating to physical, emotional, mental and spiritual energies. The smaller chakras are located where bones, joints and secondary nerve plexuses meet. They are a network through which the body, mind and spirit interact. The first three chakras deal with the physical, emotional and intellectual realms. The last four focus on the spiritual planes. The seven chakras are:

- **Muladhara:** The root chakra, found between the pubic bone and the base of the spine and associated with the gonads, is the seat of the physical body and is emotionally connected to basic issues of survival, such as food, shelter and security; it spins at the frequency of the colour red.
- **Swadhistana:** Located near the lumbo-sacral plexus, behind and below the navel, the second chakra corresponds to the reproductive glands (the ovaries and prostate), and is the centre of the emotional body, where feelings towards one's self, sexuality and others are felt; the colour of this chakra is orange.

- **Manipura:** The third chakra, found at the solar plexus in the V formed by the ribs, below the chest and above the navel, is related to the adrenal glands and the spleen, and is the seat of the mental body, where thinking and gut feelings occur; yellow is the colour frequency of this chakra.
- **Anahata:** The fourth chakra, located at the brachial plexus midway between the two breasts, is called the heart chakra (associated with the thymus gland, sometimes called the *high heart*), and is the home of the astral body, considered to be the bridge between the physical and spiritual planes; it deals with issues of unconditional love, health, healing, acceptance and forgiveness; the colour of this chakra is green.
- **Vishudda:** The next chakra, related to the parathyroid and thyroid glands, is found at the base of the throat, and is the aetheric body, concerned with speaking one's personal truth, clear communication and creative expression; the colour frequency of vishudda is blue.
- **Ajna:** The sixth chakra, commonly called the *third eye,* is located between the eyebrows and connected to the pineal gland; it is the celestial body and is related to clarity of thought and sight, as the opening of this chakra allows for broader vision and perspective, such as a flying eagle's panoramic view of the world; purple is the colour of this chakra, and it is interesting to note that the Pope and members of royalty commonly wear this colour.
- **Sahasrara:** The last chakra is the crown chakra, found just above the crown of the head; it is the ketheric body, and the gland associated with this chakra is the pituitary gland; issues of unity consciousness and interconnectedness with all things comprise the seventh chakra, which is the place of *samadhi,* or enlightenment; the coulor frequency is white.

The ancient chakra system is another way of understanding and connecting to the intelligence of the body, mind and spirit. In each yoga pose a variety of chakras are stimulated, leading to a balanced flow of energy throughout all systems and feelings of well-being.

Pranayama: Control of Breath

Pranayama is the fourth limb of yoga. It is likened to the leaves of the tree of yoga, which mingle with the air and filtrate the entire tree with prana. Through specific breathing exercises, the breath is regulated and controlled. Control of the breath consists of regulating the length and duration of the inhalation, the length and duration of the exhalation, and the retention (pauses) of the breath.

In Sanskrit, *prana* is the cosmic energy that manifests in the breath. *Ayama* means expansion, increase. So pranayama is the process in which the prana is developed and strengthened in the body, purifying the nervous system and increasing the person's vital life energy.

As a direct result, the mind also becomes calmer and more focused. It is the combination of asana and pranayama that readies the individual for deeper levels of concentration and consciousness by refining and strengthening the nervous system and the body's subtle energy.

Pratyahara: Withdrawal of the Senses

The next limb of yoga is *pratyahara.* It is the bark of the tree of yoga, which protects the tree, insulating it from the outside elements and enabling the inner energy to flow unimpeded. As the mind begins to calm and the attention settles, an inward focus is possible, no longer distracted by external events. The sense organs (eyes, ears, nose, mouth, skin) draw in from the periphery to the core to observe the inner world.

Pratyahara occurs when you are so totally absorbed in an activity that you become unaware of outside stimulation. You could be in the middle of Piccadilly Circus without seeing, hearing, smelling, feeling or tasting anything.

Immersed in a yoga pose, you become totally focused on the breath and the internal actions of the pose. Athletes commonly call this state 'being in the zone'. Here, the process of self-discovery and evolution, with the body as the experimental laboratory, continues at a more refined level.

Dharana: Concentration

This ability to focus without distraction leads to the next limb of yoga, called *dharana*. Dharana is the sap of the tree of yoga, carrying the energy and the concentration deeper inside the individual. Dharana is the one-pointed, steady focus of the mind on one object at a time. Extended periods of concentration lead to meditation.

Dhyana: Meditation

Meditation, or *dhyana,* is the seventh limb of yoga. It is the flowers of the tree of yoga, the blooming of the focused mind. Dhyana is the uninterrupted flow of concentration. This is different from the previous stage of dharana, as the ability to focus has been honed to the point where the concentration lasts for prolonged periods of time, without the one-pointed focus. Instead, the focus is expanded throughout the individual's consciousness. The mind has grown quiet, thoughts are at a minimum, and the experience is one of stillness.

Our minds are constantly fragmented and scattered, so is it any wonder that it seems impossible to focus on one object? We are accustomed to doing more than one thing at a time (for example, listening to music while we drive, or talking on the phone while preparing a meal).

Samadhi: Enlightenment

The last limb of Yoga is *samadhi.* It is the fruit of the tree of yoga, the harvest or reward of dedicated yoga practice. Samadhi has been variously described as a state of ecstasy, enlightenment and a transcending of everyday reality, where the meditator experiences a connection with the Divine and an interconnectedness with all living beings. It occurs when the individual merges with the object and there is no sense of separation between them. This is a state of peace and completion, expanded awareness and compassion with detachment (being *in* the world but not *of* it). Have you experienced moments of ecstasy, flashes of insight and knowingness, which go beyond our smaller, daily lives? Those moments are a taste of samadhi.

CHAPTER 5

Hatha Yoga and Its Many Styles

Most yoga taught in the Western world is a form of Hatha Yoga, which is comprised of physical postures, breathing techniques, relaxation and meditation. Hatha Yoga is the umbrella under which most of the sub-specialties of yoga fall. What makes the styles different from each other is their emphasis and technique.

Iyengar Yoga

Iyengar Yoga is named for Mr Iyengar, an Indian yoga master who is one of the world's most influential yogis. Iyengar Yoga focuses on precise alignment, posture and attention to subtle details. As a result, the pace of the class is slower, as poses are held for longer periods of time and repeated several times.

Standing poses are emphasized for beginners, because they set the foundation and build correct alignment from the feet up. Expect to learn a lot about your feet, shoulders, hips, pelvis and hands. When the student has reached a certain level of mastery, the study of the breath, called *pranayama,* can begin.

Iyengar Yoga uses equipment such as belts, blocks, blankets, bolsters and chairs to assist students and to help balance the body while in the pose. The use of equipment helps students achieve the best pose possible, with the maximum benefit, while minimizing the risk of injury. The equipment provides support, allowing the student to find the balance between ease and effort in a pose, breathe more freely, and go deeper into the pose. Mr Iyengar is also known for his deep knowledge and use of yoga for therapeutic purposes. The training of an Iyengar teacher is rigorous and challenging. Teachers must meet specific requirements to receive Iyengar certification.

Viniyoga

Viniyoga is a gentle-flowing, therapeutic yoga practice created by T.K.V. Desikachar of India, who developed this style based upon the teachings and philosophy of his father, Sri Krishnamacharya. One of Desikachar's students, Gary Kraftsow, recently wrote a wonderful book on Viniyoga, called *Yoga for Wellness.*

Viniyoga is a method for developing an integrated practice for each person as they grow and change through their lives. The method emphasizes flowing, modified yoga postures specific to the individual's needs to enhance healing, flexibility and stability of joints, as well as to create strength and feelings of well-being. Yoga philosophy is interwoven with practice. Frequently, it is taught privately for therapeutic purposes.

Emphasis is on breath coordinated with movement. The inhalations and exhalations and the ratio between exhalation and inhalation are morw timed as to their length and modification of classic postures, than they are in Iyengar Yoga. For example, many Viniyoga poses slightly bend the legs where Iyengar Yoga would extend them.

Ashtanga Yoga

Ashtanga Yoga is a dynamic, fast-paced, challenging series of sequential poses linked together by *ujjayi* breath (a specific breathing technique that sounds like that of Darth Vader) and a flow of postures called *vinyasas*. It is a heat-producing, detoxifying, and flowing practice that creates strength and flexibility and increases stamina.

K. Pattabhi Jois is the Indian master whose students have brought the practice all over the world. It is a style that appeals to athletically inclined individuals who enjoy intense and challenging exercise. The system is based on six series, each increasing in difficulty.

Sivananda Yoga

Sivananda Yoga is based on the teachings of Swami Sivananda of Rishikesh, India. The main focus is on yoga postures (asana), breathing (pranayama), relaxation (savasana or corpse pose), diet (vegetarian), positive thinking (vedanta) and meditation (dhyana).

There are more than 80 centres around the world. Sivanananda Yoga consists of 12 basic yoga postures to increase strength and flexibility, chanting, breath work and meditation.

Bihar Yoga

Bihar Yoga (also known as Satyananda Yoga)is based on the teachings of Swami Satyananda. Here, the main focus is on a subtle, gentle, meditative way of teaching yoga, starting with a simple series of small movements of hands, feet, wrists, ankles etc. When the student has eased into this series, he or she is then taught the classical asyanas, with the emphasis on meditation, cleansing and breathing exercises.

 Yoga is being introduced into all sorts of professions and jobs, from professional rugby and football to sedentary careers such as publishing and marketing. In each case, managemant, coaches and staff have agreed on ther benefits of practising yoga as part of an everyday routine.

Power Yoga

An Americanized hybrid of Ashtanga Yoga is *Power Yoga,* a term originating from Beryl Bender Birch, Ashtanga Yoga teacher and author of *Power Yoga.* Most power yoga is a vigorous, flowing series of postures based upon the Ashtanga Yoga system. Some health clubs have embraced Power Yoga as a transition from aerobics to yoga.

Bikram Yoga

Bikram Yoga is a challenging, hot, and aggressive yoga style developed by Bikram Choudhury. The practice consists of a prescribed sequence of 26 yoga postures designed to enhance the efficient functioning of every body system. The yoga studio is heated up to encourage sweating and the release of impurities.

People who are already in good shape, with minimal chronic ailments or injuries, are good candidates for Bikram Yoga. It is a practice designed to encourage the cleansing of the body, the releasing of toxins and maximum flexibility.

There is a yoga style for everyone, and there is some overlap between styles. As you go through life and its many transitions, you may find a need to change the style of yoga to suit where you are at that time. What worked when you were 25 may not be appropriate when you are 45.

Kripalu Yoga

Kripalu Yoga was developed by Amrit Desai, a disciple of Kripalvananda, who was an Indian Kundalini master, and is based in the USA. The three stages of Kripalu Yoga include conscious focus on alignment and breath; will and surrender through holding of postures to the edge and beyond, deepening awareness of the inner world of emotions and thought patterns; and meditation in motion, and a complete surrender and trust in the body's wisdom to hold the posture and release unnecessary blocks and tension while in a meditative state.

Namaste is a familiar greeting in yoga circles. A yoga teacher may bow her head, bring her hands into prayer position at the heart, and say namaste to the class. This is simply a way of greeting and appreciating another person. Namaste means 'the highest or the best in me salutes or greets the highest or the best in you'.

Phoenix Rising Yoga Therapy

Phoenix Rising Yoga Therapy is a blend of psychotherapeutic techniques and Kripalu Yoga, created by Michael Lee. The yoga therapist works one on one with a client and assists and holds the clients in postures, facilitating emotional and physical release.

Integral Yoga

Integral Yoga was originated by Sri Swami Satchidananda in 1966. He greatly inspired the hippie generation and increased yoga's popularity.

Integral Yoga classes are traditional, gentle Hatha Yoga classes focusing on a prescribed sequence of postures, breathing techniques, chanting, relaxation and meditation. They begin with asana practice, followed by deep relaxation, pranayama and meditation.

Ananda Yoga

Developed by J. Donald Walters (Swami Kriyananda) and inspired by Paramahansa Yogananada, Ananda Yoga is a gentle style that prepares you for meditation. Affirmations are associated with postures, and conscious attention directs the body's energy to different parts of the body. Each posture is used to increase self-awareness and self-knowledge. Students are encouraged to relax deeply into postures.

ISHTA Yoga (Yoga Zone)

ISHTA (Integrated Science of Hatha, Tantra and Ayurveda) was created by Alan Finger and his father. ISHTA Yoga classes combine Ashtanga Yoga with the precision of Iyengar Yoga, breathing practices and meditation.

Anusara Yoga

Anusara Yoga is based upon Hatha Yoga and biomechanical principles. It is physically grounding and focuses upon inner and outer alignment, while keeping the heart open and flowing with grace through the postures. John Friend, the founder, says Anusara Yoga differs from other Hatha Yogas because of its three main principles:

- **Attitude:** There is an opening to grace with and to one's own true nature.
- **Alignment:** Each pose is done with an integrated awareness of all different parts of the body.
- **Action:** Each pose is performed with a heart-centred focus and a balance between muscular stability and expansive inner freedom.

Kundalini Yoga

Kundalini is a Tantric Yoga discipline, brought to the West by Yogi Bhajan, based upon the arousal of the *kundalini* (serpent power) energy housed in the base of the spine. Powerful breathing techniques combined with specific yoga postures and chanting are designed to awaken the kundalini from the base of the spine, where it will travel through the major energy centres of the subtle body, resulting in spiritual transformation and unity consciousness.

Finding the Type of Yoga That's Right for You

Yoga is a very rich and varied tradition that is alive and constantly evolving to meet the needs of individuals. It rewards those who devote themselves to the practice with vibrant health and well-being. The yoga styles described in this chapter are not an exhaustive list of the many types taught in the UK and USA today. However, they are a useful guide to the person seeking the yoga that fits his lifestyle.

The type of yoga you choose depends upon why you want to practice. For example, someone who is inflexible, with tight hamstrings and a tight lower back, may want to create more flexibility and space within his body. The primary goal is to increase physical comfort and range of motion. Another person may feel extremely stressed, with symptoms such as headaches and lower back tightness, and may want to find a yoga class that focuses on relaxation, breathing, and meditation techniques as a way to manage stress and tension. Another person may be recovering from illness or surgery and be interested in a class where passive yoga postures are taught. And yet another person may want to be very active and challenged in yoga class, sweating, building strength and developing a leaner body.

Sample several different classes until you find one that satisfies your needs. Decide why you want to try yoga. What do you want to get out of the experience? The teacher is a most important factor in your decision.

Ask the teacher for her credentials and background. The match between student and teacher is crucial. After attending a class, ask yourself:

- Did I receive attentive guidance from the teacher, or did I have to look around the class and imitate the other students?
- Do I feel a little sore from using my body differently, or did I actually get injured in class?
- Am I feeling energized and calm, or frustrated and stressed out?
- Was the class small enough for me to get the amount of individualized attention I want?
- Did I feel comfortable and at ease?
- Were the teacher's instructions clear enough that I could follow and learn from them?

Numerous yoga videos are available for home practice. Some of the best videos for beginners are listed in the Resources appendix at the back of this book. Yoga retreats and holidays have also grown in popularity. Most of these are in beautiful locations in the UK and abroad, where you can immerse yourself in yoga, relax and take in the sights. They are a fabulous way to study a particular style of yoga with a teacher or two.

Videos should supplement, not replace, yoga class. It is important to receive feedback from your teacher. Otherwise, you may not know whether you are doing the poses and breath work correctly. Then you can go home and practise, practise, practise.

CHAPTER 6

Getting Started

Yoga is very user-friendly. It requires very little in the way of equipment and space. The most important part is to show up, have an open mind and be present with your self. As one of my teachers once said, the hardest part of yoga practice is rolling out the mat.

Attitude Is Everything

Yoga is all about expanding self-awareness. Therefore it is most important to listen to your body as you practise postures and breathing techniques. It is imperative to practise safely in a non-aggressive manner. When opening up tight areas in the body that are unaccustomed to stretching, you may feel discomfort. This discomfort may be due to stiff joints, tight muscles or tightness of *fascia* (the fibrous inter-connective tissue that is like a web between skin and muscle and also encases organs).

Breathing into the area will help ease the initial distress. Continuous breathing is the key. Often, shortness or holding breath is a very good indication that you are working too hard or thinking too much. Let your breath inform and infuse your practice. Yoga is yoga because the breath is connected with the continuum of getting into the posture, being in the posture and coming out of the posture. It is this connection of conscious movement with conscious breath that differentiates yoga poses from other physical disciplines such as gymnastics or dance.

The time you spend doing yoga is a sacred, intimate time when you learn about, accept, and nurture yourself. Try to schedule time for yoga every day, even if it is only 10 to 15 minutes. Then your practice will become part of your daily routine, integrated with your lifestyle.

Yoga is an internally motivated practice. Comparing oneself to another practitioner or to a picture in a book, and trying to mould your body into this ideal pose is not useful. We are all different, and we come with bodies of all shapes and sizes and special needs. One person may be able to perform a backbend with ease and look beautiful doing it, but she might struggle with forward bends. Modification of poses is always possible and encouraged. This is where we begin to have reverence for the body and compassion for ourselves. Then the true meaning of the yoga is felt. Yoga puts you on the path of self-exploration where you begin to trust what you feel and believe.

A quiet, well-ventilated, comfortably warm room keeps the muscles supple. If the room is too warm, it will be distracting, causing either irritation or lethargy. A hardwood floor is terrific, but firm carpeting will also work fine. Clothing should be comfortable for full range of movement. T-shirts, leggings and shorts are appropriate yoga gear. Yoga is done barefoot to tactilely feel, sense and ground the feet.

There is a difference between pain and feeling the intensity of an action. Don't force or strain when performing the poses. Strive for a balance between ease and effort. You should feel better after yoga, although some soreness is normal. Soreness is healthy pain, while searing, persistent pain is unhealthy, indicating injury. Any injury, of course, should be treated by a health professional.

Yoga Equipment

Some styles of yoga use a variety of equipment to help the body attain good alignment, balance and ease in a pose. This enables you to perform a posture without tiring, thus allowing a longer duration in the pose without strain, and give you the maximum benefit. The use of such equipment helps to open the inner body while supporting muscular effort and minimizing strain and excessive striving in a pose. People with medical problems and the elderly will find equipment invaluable in helping them practice poses that they might otherwise be unable to do.

Dr Benjamin Spock was a guru to parents for many generations. During the last years of his life, doctors told him he would never be able to walk again. Instead of resigning himself to that fate, Spock began a regimen of macrobiotics, shiatsu massage, psychoanalysis and yoga. After four yoga classes with Rama Berch, he was able to walk again.

There are many different pieces of equipment that can be used to enhance your practice. They can be purchased through catalogues and at some yoga centres. Below is a list of simple equipment, some of which may already be part of your household:

- **Yoga mat:** this is a useful non-slip mat that provides traction and grip so you can concentrate on doing the posture without worrying about slipping.
- **Strap or belt:** a strap has many uses, for example, stretching the hamstrings in a variety of poses, or making a 'longer arm' to hold onto for shoulder-opening exercises.
- **Three firm cotton or woollen blankets:** blankets are handy for sitting on, and for placing under knees, heads and torsos for headstands and shoulderstands.
- **Metal or wooden chair without arms:** a chair is wonderful for supported and modified poses.
- **Wooden or foam block or phone book:** this comes in handy for 'bringing the floor to you' in many postures (for example, if you are in a standing forward bend and your hands don't reach the floor, a block placed under each hand eases the effort and stretch in the hamstrings); an old phone book can be encased in strong tape (gaffer or duct tape works well).
- **Empty wall space:** a wall is a very useful tool that reinforces correct alignment, symmetry and balance.

What are *mudras?*

Mudras are specific ways of holding the hands, the fingers and body to represent specific acts of offering and saluting, and to produce certain energetic effects, targeting the energy to specific areas and developing energy circuits in the body. They affect how we experience postures and the breath.

CHAPTER 7

Breathing Basics

The breath is the vehicle for *prana*, the vital life force. It is the universal energy that sustains all life. The prana enters the body upon inhalation, supplying every cell with energy, oxygen and nutrients. With exhalation, waste and toxins are released. The breath is the bridge between the physical and spiritual worlds.

The Anatomy of the Breath

The lungs are not made of muscle tissue, but they have elasticity and can receive the actions of surrounding muscles. The lungs must depend upon muscular action for their expansion and contraction.

It is the diaphragm, the intercostals (the muscles located between the ribs) and the abdominal muscles that play a key role in breathing. The diaphragm, located in the chest, is a large umbrella-shaped muscle that is responsible for 75 per cent of the work. It attaches to the top of the *sternum* (the breastbone), the middle and lower ribs and to the first, second, third and fourth lumbar vertebrae of the lower spine. Under the diaphragm lie the abdominal organs, and above it the heart and lungs.

With inhalation, the diaphragm comes down towards the abdomen and expands, making room for the incoming breath. Upon exhalation, the diaphragm rises up to release the air. As the lungs expand with the inhalation, the abdomen expands, the intercostal muscles lengthen and spread laterally, and the top chest (the part near the collarbone) expands and broadens.

This entire process is reversed during exhalation. The breath is squeezed out of the stomach, the ribs and intercostal muscles contract, and the breath is pushed out of the body.

Yogic Breathing

When you begin practising yoga, your respiration may be shallow, with small, fairly rapid breaths. The average person breathes 16 to 18 breaths per minute. As you continue your yoga practice, your rate of breath will become slower, and each inhalation and exhalation will become longer and fuller. Deeper breaths allow the energy to reach every cell.

The yoga postures open the body to receive the breath, resulting in increased elasticity of the lungs and *intercostal muscles* (located between the ribs). Forward bends stretch the back of the body and fill the back of the lungs; backbends open the front of the body and the front of the lungs; and lateral bends lengthen the sides of the body and the space between the ribs (the intercostal muscles). Inversions bring greater oxygen and blood flow to the brain.

In yoga, the body is considered to be a container for the life force. The nervous system is the electrical circuitry, which conducts the energy of the body. The spinal column, called *sushumna*, is the central pathway. Two other main pathways are the *pingala*, to the right of the sushumna, and the *ida*, on the left side. Balance between the ida and pingala increases the energy flow to the sushumna. The ida channel cools the body and corresponds to the parasympathetic nervous system, while the pingala heats up the body and is the sympathetic nervous system. These main channels correspond to the central nervous system and are called *nadis*. There are thousands of smaller nadis comprising the peripheral nervous system. When the energy in the body increases significantly, it is said that the *kundalini* (serpent power) energy rises up the spine (the sushumna), opening the various energy centres in the body and causing spiritual evolution within the individual.

Yoga links the breath to the body. The breath is the bridge between mind and matter, between body and spirit. During inhalation, we are receiving life. Upon exhaling, we are returning what we don't need and ridding the body-mind of impurities.

Yogic breathing is almost always done through the nostrils. The nose is a complex and extremely efficient filtering system of foreign particles. As the breath enters the nostrils, it is moistened and warmed to body temperature. Breathing through the nose allows for deeper, fuller and more controllable breathing.

Mouth breathing is for those times of athletic competition, such as sprint running, when the body is in oxygen deprivation, due to the excessive demands being placed upon it. Then mouth breathing becomes the last resort. For these reasons, it is considered a waste of energy to breathe through the mouth.

Breathing Exercises

Breathing is an important part of yoga. Try the following breathing exercises as a part of your yoga practice.

Complete Breath

Lie down with bent knees, and begin breathing through your nostrils and observing your breath. Become aware of the natural length of your inhalation and exhalation, and the pauses in between. Remain relaxed, without changing or forcing the breath. Let the breath flow smoothly and evenly. Relax your facial muscles and jaw.

Place your hands on your lower abdomen, allowing them to rest there lightly. As you breathe in, feel your hands fill with your breath as your stomach gently expands. Note how your stomach contracts, moving away from your hands and receding into your body upon exhalation. Spend 10 to 12 breaths observing the movement of the breath in your stomach.

Next, lightly place your palms on your lower, front floating ribs. Let your wrists relax down to your body. Again, let the breath come into your hands upon inhalation and feel your ribs contracting on exhalation. Do this for another 10 to 12 breaths.

Last, place your hands on the collarbone and observe the breath filling the area under your hands on the inhalation. Notice how your top chest recedes with the exhalation. Practise this for 10 to 12 breaths.

Holding your breath to get it to the 'right' rhythm is harmful and unnecessary. In young children, the breath becomes a whole body action. The body fills fully, easily, silently and without inhibition. In yoga, the breath must be just like a baby's breath.

Then allow your arms to come back to your sides, palms facing up. Continue to watch your breath, feeling the three-part breathing pattern. You may find that the breath comes in more easily to one area than it does to another. With practice, you will be able to breathe more fully and deeply, filling your entire body with the breath.

Raising the Arms with the Breath

Stand with your feet directly under your hips. Plant your feet firmly on the floor and lengthen up through your legs and your spine, to the top of your head. Keep your arms at your sides, palms facing forwards. Begin normal, relaxed breathing through the nostrils.

As you inhale, raise your arms slowly away from your sides, feeling your stomach fill up, then feeling your ribs expand and the top of your chest broaden with the breath. Let your expanding stomach, chest and ribs help you reach your arms up. At the top of the inhalation, your arms will be over your head. When exhalation naturally starts, press your palms down as you watch the breath leave the top chest, and squeeze out of the lungs and the stomach. Allow the pressing down of your palms to help push the breath out of your body. Practice coordinating lifting and lowering the arms with the flow of the breath.

Do at least five breaths this way. Be aware of how you feel after this experience. Do you feel more grounded and internally connected? Are you calmer and more focused?

This breathing exercise is a wonderful way to learn about your breath and is also excellent for opening and warming up the body. Don't worry if your inhalation is finished before the breath reaches the top chest. With practice, your exhalation will become longer, and this will positively affect the length of the inhalation.

Strengthening the Diaphragm

The diaphragm is a large and powerful muscle involved in the respiration process. Like any muscle, it needs to be exercised in order for it to become strong and function optimally.

Lie on your back and place a 4.5kg (10lb) sandbag (or bag of rice or flour) on your abdomen, just below the floating ribs. Then lie back and breathe normally, without force or strain, for five minutes. Don't try to lift the bag with your breathing. Let the breath touch the bag. If you feel fatigued before five minutes have passed, lessen the duration of the exercise.

You will feel the weight of the bag as your chest rises and falls, but do not try to consciously lift the bag. Let your breath and the bag exercise your diaphragm muscle. A strong, not tense, diaphragm muscle will lead to fuller, deeper and more efficient breathing, and will also aid in the pumping and circulating of the lymphatic system.

After five minutes, take the bag off the diaphragm and continue to observe your breath. You may notice a difference. Practise bag breathing for five minutes a day, gradually building up to 10 minutes. Do this for a month, scheduling yourself for three days of practice and then one day off. Observe the changes. Your breathing will deepen and become more efficient and the diaphragm will be stronger. This exercise can be repeated at any time to exercise and strengthen the diaphragm.

Coordinating Breath with Movement

When the breath is coordinated with the movement, less physical effort is required in a pose. The breath linked with the movement supplies the vital energy necessary to move through the pose with ease.

In general, the inhalation is done while creating extension and expansion in the body. This is the preparation for the pose. Most movement into a pose is performed upon exhalation. Elongating the front of the body will encourage inhalation, while curling and shortening the front body will invite exhalation. The exhalation also contracts the abdominals, which provide support and stability for the lower back. Coming down into a pose is done on the exhalation, and coming up out of a pose is done on the inhalation. Continuous breathing is vital, regardless of the synchronization with the movement.

Pay Attention to Your Breathing

Observe your breath during the day. Check in with your breath every hour at a specified time. Slow down and tune into the quality and length of the inhalation, exhalation and pauses in between. Note whether the breath is smooth or ragged, shallow

Take several breaths through your nostrils and then through your mouth, observing the differences. Was the length of the inhalation and exhalation the same? Does your mouth feel dry as a result of breathing through the mouth? Which style feels more comfortable? Initially, breathing through the nostrils may be difficult.

CHAPTER 8
The Asanas

Asanas are a vital part of yoga. The postures are more than physical exercises. They clean, control and discipline the mind and the body; sharpen the natural intelligence; and awaken every cell in the body. The many different types of asanas help tone, balance and stimulate every part of the body.

What Are Asanas?

Yoga is a process of learning to recognize and observe the reactions and habitual patterns of the mind, body and breath. When you become aware of your patterns, you can slowly, diligently, exchange them for new, more balanced patterns of movement, breathing and thinking.

The asanas are geometric, each with their own form and shape. In any pose, there must be a clear action, sense of direction and centre of gravity. In order to maintain the centre of gravity, the muscles must be properly aligned. Stability of the pelvic and shoulder girdles is essential to the balance and symmetry of the spine.

In every pose, for every action, there is an equal opposing reaction. Moving in one direction won't create positive change in the body. There cannot be extension without foundation. In every pose, there is a foundation from which extension is possible. This foundation creates the stability and space in the joints, the lengthening of muscle, and the suppleness and correct placement of the organs.

In standing poses, the feet are rooted down, allowing the legs and the spine to lengthen and extend away from the feet. The buttock bones are the foundation in seated poses from which the spine lifts and elongates. In inverted postures, the head, hands or forearms provide the foundation and stability from which the torso and legs lengthen.

Remember that the goal is not the pose itself. It is the meditative process from beginning to end, which includes reflection on the effects of the asana. The asanas create different effects:

· Standing poses enhance vitality
· Seated poses are calming
· Twists are cleansing
· Supine poses are restful
· Prone poses are energizing
· Inverted postures increase mental strength
· Balancing poses create lightness

- Backbends are exhilarating
- Jumping develops agility

The Importance of Practice

Practice and repetition of the asanas align the bones, joints and muscles, producing strength and flexibility, balanced muscle action, stamina and endurance. It is through analysis of action, by trial and error, that right effort is discovered. Right effort allows a balance between ease and effort in a pose. Then proper stretching and contracting of muscle groups are possible, the bones stack and feed into the joints, and the nervous system is soothed. Meditation in motion then occurs.

Benefits from practice are cumulative over time. Practice should be systematic, beginning with basic postures and, over time, integrating more complex asanas into your sequence. Repeating the pose two or three times is important for gaining knowledge about the body in relation to the pose.

In general, it takes about two years to become familiar and comfortable with the poses. Initially, great progress may be made, due to the disciplining of the grosser movements of the body. Slower growth is apparent as you begin to refine and get into the subtleties of each asana. This is where the real learning takes place. Patience, perseverance, openness and effort are the keys to a successful practice. Practice positively changes the physical as well as the mental, emotional and spiritual states.

It is important to understand that the asana is not the final pose. The asana is a continuum of mindfully setting up for the pose, coming into the pose, and carefully coming out of the pose. The pose is constantly evolving. It is not static.

Attention to accuracy and appropriate adjustment while in the pose is essential. If you set up well for the posture, then the posture will be optimal and most beneficial. The energy will flow evenly. If you come out of the pose with awareness, the risk of injury and jarring the nervous system is minimal.

The frequency of practice is an individual matter. Schedule your yoga time into your busy routine, because regular practice is important. Some people may feel great satisfaction and benefit from a weekly yoga session, while others may thrive on a daily practice or two to three times a week. This depends upon your needs, time constraints and motivation. Remember that a little bit can go a long way. Doing a few poses at a time frequently may be better for you than practising for two hours at a time.

Asanas can be done at any time of the day. When you practise in the morning, the body tends to be stiffer, but the mind is sharper. In an evening yoga session, the body is suppler, but the mind is duller.

Keep the eyes soft but open as you practise. Your eyes will gaze externally but their focus will be internal, scanning the body for feedback. Your ears will listen to the soft and natural sound of your breath, ensuring that you *are* breathing in a smooth and continuous manner. Your mouth should remain closed.

Many poses and breathing techniques in yoga are therapeutic. In certain conditions, however, specific poses are contraindicated (not recommended). They are:

· **Cardiac disorders:** do not put your arms over your head.
· **Menstruation:** do not perform inversions.
· **Pregnancy:** do not practise breath retention.
· **Glaucoma or eye problems, ear pain or congestion:** don't practise breath retention or inversions.
· **Hypertension:** do not practise breath retention or inverted poses, except for the legs-up-the-wall pose.

If you have any condition or disorder, or are pregnant, check with your doctor before beginning yoga. Any questions or concerns should be brought to the attention of a qualified yoga teacher for clarification.

Your stomach should be empty when practising asanas. A useful guideline is to wait two hours after a light meal and four hours after a heavy meal, before you practise yoga. The asanas stretch, compress, twist and invert the abdominal area. Sensations of stomach distress, such as nausea, heartburn or cramp, could result from practising on a full stomach.

The Value of Yoga Classes

Attending yoga classes with a teacher can enhance your yoga practice. It is important for your understanding and growth to be observed by a teacher who can provide feedback about your practice. Very often, we think we are doing correct action in our poses, but there are misalignments and unawareness that can detract from the precision and benefits of the pose. Having someone's eyes upon you, and his careful guidance, can increase your awareness and stimulate your self-knowledge.

The teacher may challenge your way of being in a pose and suggest new actions, which will enhance and deepen your practice. Subtleties you might never have thought of can become known to you. Then you can go back home recharged and motivated, and practise with this new-found awareness.

The group energy of a class, plus being in community with like-minded individuals, can enhance your experience of yoga. You can share experiences with class members and help increase each other's awareness and knowledge.

The *Yoga Sutras* say that the asanas must have the dual qualities of alertness and relaxation, and be comfortable and steady. When you begin yoga, everything is an effort. The body-mind system is navigating through foreign territory, assuming totally new ways of moving and being. Eventually, effort and ease are balanced in asana practice, and the breath flows smoothly.

Principles of Action and Anatomy

There are several key actions consistently performed in yoga asanas. A brief discussion of anatomy will help you understand the mechanics of the body.

The Importance of Foundation

The rooting of the foundation, or base, allows extension, space, balance and ease in a pose. If you're looking for proof, sit down on a firm chair with your heels directly under your hips and your shoulders over your hips. First sit in a slouched position and note how that feels and be aware of the quality of your breath. Now sit up tall, without leaning against the chair back. Press your buttock bones (the bony protuberances you sit on), into the chair seat. Observe the rebounding, lengthening action that lifts your spine out of the pelvis. Enhance this by lengthening up through the top of your head. Observe the quality of the breath. Is it fuller and deeper than when you sat in a slumped position?

Hugging Muscle to Bone

The function of muscle is to support the skeletal system. This cannot occur if muscle does not actively adhere to the bone. If muscle is not supporting bone, then the bone cannot stay in its socket. The joints are then not properly supported. This situation has a domino effect throughout the body, underlining the necessity of drawing muscle energy into the bone to create good alignment and integrity.

The hugging muscle action occurs when we draw the muscle in to the bone. This creates support for the bone, lengthens the muscle and draws the bone into the socket, where it belongs.

Have you seen very flexible people who walk as if their bones are not connected? They need to build strength to support their joints and to hold their bones in the right place. Over-stiff people need to break down some of the strength to create more space and flexibility. However, they are already supporting their joints much more than the over- flexible person.

People who begin yoga with stiffness bemoan the fact that they are inflexible. They tend to look enviously at their loose classmates, who seem to be able to effortlessly ease in and out of postures. However, it is much easier to break down stiffness than to build up muscle strength. And flexible people tend to get injured more frequently because their support system is not in place. So in some ways, it is better to be stiff with support than flexible without support.

The good news is that yoga is the great equalizer. The poses will develop flexibility and strength where they are needed. Careful attention and practice while in the poses will help correct these problems over time, resulting in better alignment, a balance of strength and flexibility in the muscles, and integrity of the leg joints.

Practise this: stand with your feet wider apart than your hips. Place your hands on your hips. Press down into your feet and draw the inner thighs away from each other. Observe the hugging muscle action in the thighs as they draw into the bone. This exercise can also be done standing in a doorway and pressing the outside of the feet against the doorjamb while doing the above actions. Don't your legs feel more solid and stable?

Shoulder Blades and Arms

The job of the shoulder blades is to open the chest and support the upper body. This is very important, as the heart and lungs are housed there, and they need proper space to function well. And when the chest is open and supported, the breath can fully enter the lungs.

In order to do this, the shoulder blades must press into the body, and the muscles surrounding them must actively work and contract to keep the shoulder blades flush with the upper back. Move the shoulder blades so they feel as if they are moving down the back toward the waist. This action will naturally lift the chest. The muscles around the upper side ribs also have to hug the body to provide length and support. It takes time and practice to strengthen these muscles, especially if they are only accustomed to stretching.

When a person's upper back is rounded, that is an indication that the shoulder blades are off the back, providing no support. The head may lean forward, placing excessive demands on the neck and upper back muscles, while the chest caves in and the shoulders roll forward, and the arms are forward in the socket. The arms and shoulder blades are disconnected from the upper body, and the breath tends to be short and shallow.

In the discussion of poses, you will be reminded to keep your shoulder blades on your back. If this is confusing, try this exercise: Lie down on your back with your knees bent. Extend your arms, with palms facing each other, up to the ceiling. Stretch your fingertips up to the ceiling.

Observe how the shoulder blades are now off the back and the arms are also disconnected from the shoulder sockets. Now draw your upper arm bone down to the floor while stretching out through the fingertips. Feel the shoulder blades press onto the floor. Continue stretching into the fingers as you bring the blades to the floor.

This is the dynamic, opposing stretch you want in your arms – going in equally opposing directions, stretching expansively out from the centre of the body into the fingertips and back into the core of the body, with the arms in the socket and the shoulder blades supporting the upper body. Practice this daily, doing 10 or 20 repetitions, to build up the strength of the upper back muscles.

Maintaining Extension in the Spine

There must be space between the spinal vertebrae to create a healthy and supple spine. A long spine allows the nerves sufficient room to exit from the spinal cord. Impingement on the nerves can cause nerve pain and damage. Extension of the spine affects every system in the body – —the nervous system, the circulatory system, the respiratory system, the digestive system and the endocrine system.

When we do poses, we inhale to prepare for the pose and to create expansion in the body and length in the spine. Then we are ready to safely do the pose. Remember that is the grounding action in any pose that allows the extension.

The extension of the spine also creates the freedom for opening, broadness of the upper body (chest and upper back), and the spaciousness of the pelvis (the lower back and lower abdomen). Internal space means that the organs have room to do their work and enough room for the breath to enter the cells, bones, organs and all the places in between.

Spinal Curves

The spine has four natural curves, running from front to back, which are designed to absorb the shocks and jolts to the body during daily activities such as running, walking and sitting in a car. The *cervical* (neck) spine is concave, the *thoracic* (upper back) spine is slightly convex, the *lumbar* (lower back) spine is concave, and the coccyx is convex. Any deviation from the normal curves can cause pain, dysfunction and disease.

One of the goals in asana practice is to maintain the natural curves of the spine. We do not want to flatten out the neck or lower back, round the middle back too much, or create *swayback* (excessive lower-back concavity) or shortening of the neck by lifting the chin or jutting it forward.

What is scoliosis?

An abnormal curve of the spine from side to side, with one side becoming contracted while the other side is long. According to Mary Pullig Schatz, MD, *functional scoliosis* is a curve that is caused by conditions, such as asymmetrical work, differences in leg length and back spasms.

Because the spine is attached to the arms, legs and chest by the shoulder and pelvic girdles and ribs, with the head balanced on top of the spine, every movement affects the spine, and vice versa. For example, if the shoulder joints are inflexible, you may compensate by overarching your lower back when your arms are raised in an activity. This places excessive strain on the lower back and can cause problems in time.

If the hips are stiff, with little range of movement, the pelvic area will be unable to move fluidly and freely. This distortion will be transferred upwards throughout the spine and the body. Various muscle groups can affect the curve of the lower back. They are listed here.

Paraspinals

The paraspinals are deep muscles on either side of the spine, which support the spine when it is vertical and are involved in rotating the spine, bending it backwards and sideways. If the paraspinals are too tight, swayback will occur; if they are too lax they can lead to a flat back. When the paraspinals are overworked, they can go into spasm. Yoga helps the paraspinals by stretching and strengthening them.

Hip Flexors

The hip flexors, which allow the thigh to lift, affect the stability of the lower back. Because they attach to the front of the pelvis, tight hip flexors will cause the pelvis to tilt forward, creating swayback.

Abdominal Muscles

Abdominal muscles function to support the abdominal organs and the lumbar spine. If the abdominal muscles are weak, the pelvis will drop forward, creating excessive strain and shortening of the lower back.

Psoas Muscles

The psoas muscles are extremely important muscles that affect our posture. The pair of psoas muscles, on either side of the body, attach from the groin internally, through the pelvis to the anterior lumbar spine and the diaphragm (breathing) muscle. If the psoas is tight and constricted, *lordosis,* an excessive lower back curve, can occur. A tight psoas muscle also impinges upon the internal organs located in the pelvic area, creating less space for the organs to do their work. Weakness of the psoas muscle can contribute to rounding of the lower back.

Hamstrings

The hamstrings insert onto the *ischial tuberosities* (buttock bones) and into the back of the knee. Tight hamstrings will tilt the pelvis backward and create a flattened lumbar curve.

Quadriceps

Quadricep muscles in the front of the thigh contract to allow the hamstrings to lengthen in forward-bending poses, while the hamstring muscles contract during backbends as the quadricep muscles elongate. Contraction of the quadricep muscle while lifting the kneecap sends a physiological message to the hamstrings to release.

The quadriceps and the hamstrings work together as partners in supporting the legs, pelvis and spine. They are an example of equal and opposite actions in muscular energy, which result in balanced effort. This synergistic relationship between muscle groups occurs throughout the body.

The Ribcage

The ribcage has a front, a back and two sides. Most people are only aware of their front ribs because they can see them. The ribs extend all the way up to the collarbones and down to the middle abdomen. Eight of the ribs are attached to the sternum or the spine, and four are floating ribs attached to each other. The muscles between the ribs are called intercostal muscles. They are responsible for stretching upon inhalation to allow the rib cage to expand and make room for the lungs to fill up, and to contract with the rib cage when the lungs empty.

The ribs, like the pelvis, must be in a neutral position to facilitate extension of the spine. If the front ribs are thrust forward, the back is shortened and the kidneys are compressed.

The ribs must lengthen away from the hips, to create a long spine. Space is then created between the hips and the armpits and between the ribs (as the intercostal muscles stretch). Breathing becomes deeper and fuller as a result.

Soft Stomach

In our society, there is too much emphasis on obtaining a flat stomach by sucking the stomach in. This creates tightness and hardness in the abdominal area, its organs, the diaphragm and the groins. The breath also becomes restricted and the flow of energy to the pelvis is blocked. Movement becomes restricted.

The stomach needs to remain soft and receptive. In poses, there can be a lengthening of the abdominal area by lifting the ribs away from the hips, and a slight drawing in of the lower abdomen, but this must be done without tension, through synchronization of the movement with the energy and the breath.

Soft and Spacious Pelvic Floor

Like the stomach, the pelvic floor needs to be soft and spacious, without hardening of the anal or genital area. The pelvis should be in a neutral position to maintain the correct placement of the sacrum and the natural curves of the spine. It may be helpful to visualize the pelvic area as a broad basin filled with water. If it tips too far forwards or back, the water will spill out.

The pelvis has three dimensions in which it moves: front to back, side to side and up and down. A pelvis that tilts forward increases the lumbar curve, shortens the lower back muscles and causes a swaybacked position. A backward-tilting pelvis tucks the coccyx, causes the lumbar curve to flatten and may be the result of a tight psoas muscle. A pelvis that is higher on one side, leans more to one side, or has one side further forward, also distorts the sacrum, spine and legs. The pelvis plays a crucial role in connecting the legs to the spine, which is why it is so important to have the thigh bones insert correctly into the pelvis at the right angle.

The Hips and Groin

The hips remain level to one another as much as possible, without forcing the action. Level hips balance the sacrum and a balanced sacrum balances the spine. The iliacus muscles (on the front of the hip) lengthen down, allowing the lower stomach to lift up. Then the inner body lifts and the psoas lengthens and the groin remains soft and long. Like the stomach and the pelvic floor, we want to keep the groin as soft as possible. The stomach and the groin can softly recede into the body. Hardening or pushing the groin forward shortens it, reduces the openness of the hips and contributes to lower back discomfort.

The Sacrum

The word *sacrum* means 'sacred bone'. The sacrum is a flat, triangular bone formed by the fusion of the last five spinal vertebrae. It is part of the back wall of the pelvis.

The pelvis joins the spine to the legs and the sacrum acts as the fulcrum upon which the spine rests and from which it arises. The weight transfers from the head down the spine, and then distributes through the widest part of the sacrum to the thickest part of the pelvis. Then the weight shunts forward to either the sit bones, if one is sitting, or down the femurs (thigh bones) to the feet, if one is standing. From there the feet rebound the energy back up the legs to the top of the head, allowing for extension.

The sacrum's alignment is crucial. Correct use of the feet, legs, pelvic floor and abdomen allows the downward weight to transfer and the sacrum to be balanced. Many of us do not completely transfer the weight from the sacrum to the sitting bones or the feet. The weight may stay at the sacrum, causing undue stress and strain on the vertebral discs just above the sacrum (L3, L4, L5). Indeed, many people have back injuries in this area. The natural curve of the lumbar spine (lower back) is concave. The top of the sacrum slightly tilts in to the body.

Knees

The knees are very vulnerable joints, situated between the ankles and the hips and dependent upon them for stability and alignment. The most important rule is that there should be no pain in the knees during poses. If pain should occur, the pose needs to be modified or skipped. The activity and grounding of feet, the full stretching of legs and lifting of kneecaps in straight-legged poses, ensure healthy knees by fully supporting and opening the knees.

To get the feeling of the quadricep muscle contracting and hugging the bone and the kneecap lifting, do this exercise: stand with your feet under your hips. Lift one foot off the ground and just let it dangle. Observe how difficult it is to maintain your balance when the foot and leg are dull and without energy. Now lengthen the heel and the balls of the foot away from the leg. Note the action and energy in the entire leg and foot. Pay particular attention to the upper knee and lower quadricep muscle. They are now actively engaged. This is the action we try to maintain in our straight-legged poses.

Hyperextension of the knee is a common problem that occurs when trying to straighten the leg. Unfortunately, this is a wrong action, which can result in overstretching the tendons and ligaments of the knee. Tendons and ligaments are not meant to be elastic, as their job is to provide support for the joints. The hyperextended knee is pressed back, rounding the back of the knee, overstretching the calf muscles and bypassing the space and extension in the legs.

Hyperextension of the knees distorts the alignment of the hips, pelvis and spine, and causes abnormal wear and tear on these joints. Drawing the top of the thighbone into the hip socket and pressing the neck of the big toe down will help prevent hyperextension. In order to lengthen the leg without hyperextending the knee, it is important that the quadricep muscle contracts and firms before the back of the knee stretches.

Most people who hyperextend their knees do so because their hamstrings are tight and the quadricep muscle is weak where it meets the top of the knee. When hyperextending, the shinbones do not insert properly into the knee joint. The shinbone presses back beyond the knees, overstretching the back of the knee and the calf muscles, and then the thighbone does not insert correctly into the pelvis. This affects and distorts the alignment of the leg, pelvis and spine, and never allows you to connect into your hips.

Fully Stretching the Legs

The legs must be fully opened and stretched for the spine to lengthen out of the pelvis and for the torso to have freedom of movement. Those with inflexible hamstrings often experience back pain or discomfort, due to the rounding of the upper and lower back. The tightness of the hamstrings reverberates up the body, pulling the muscles of the back down, flattening the lower back, tilting the pelvis backwards and tucking in the coccyx. If the hamstrings can be progressively stretched through yoga postures, the back muscles will release as well.

To fully stretch the legs, the feet must press down into the floor as the leg stretches up from the grounding of the feet. Remember: for every action there is an opposite and equal reaction. The lifting of the kneecap is also crucial. Lifting of the kneecap is achieved by the contraction of the quadricep muscle on the front of the thigh, where it attaches to the top of the knee. The top of the kneecap becomes imbedded in the lower quadriceps. Remember that this action helps release the hamstring muscle. Simultaneously, the thighbone draws up into the hip socket. These actions create space and extension in the legs.

Try this exercise to feel the full stretch of the leg: stand and bend your knees. Feel the weight come into your feet. Keeping the weight in your feet and pressing them down, extend from the shins to the heels, lift up the knees and lengthen the muscles from the knees to the hips, like you are pulling socks up your legs. The 'socks' are your thigh muscles. Contract the quadricep muscle before and faster than you stretch the back of the knee. Do this without pushing the knees or shins back. See how slowly you can do this, observing the stretching pull of the leg muscles as they lengthen away from each other. Also notice that the quadricep muscles are actively working and will strengthen over time from this action. Do this several times and repeat often to strengthen the quadricep and train the leg muscles to stretch fully.

The Active Yoga Foot

The foot in yoga should always be energetic and active (but not tense), unless you are in a relaxing, restorative posture. When standing, begin by spreading the toes away from each other, creating a broad base with your feet. Feel the balls and the bones of the feet spreading apart.

Stretch your toes forward as you lengthen the heels away from the toes to lengthen the feet. Press your feet down strongly, grounding the big toe and little toe mounds of the feet and the centre of the heel. Press down evenly on the inner and outer sides of the feet, and the balls and heels of the feet.

From the rooting action of the feet, lift your inner and outer arches up into the feet. The lift of the arches stimulates muscle action up your legs. If you cannot feel the arches lift, help them by lifting up your (spread) toes. These actions are performed even if the foot is not against something, as if it was pressing into an imaginary surface.

The actions of the feet create a healthy foot from which the alignment of the whole body develops. The support of the legs and pelvis are fully dependent upon the feet. The lifting of the arches is excellent for developing the arches, which support the weight of the body and rebound the energy and extension back up the body. The grounding, broadening and lengthening of the foot are equally important.

How to Work with the Postures in This Book

Read through the description and look at the photographs of the pose before doing the posture. Initially, do the pose several times for short periods of time to get familiar with the shape and actions of the posture. Remember to breathe continuously and smoothly in the pose.

Do not get discouraged if the poses seem difficult at first. This is normal. Remember: it takes time to explore your mind and body connections and change your patterns of movement and perception.

Experiment with the different ways to practise to determine which way of practising the pose will benefit you most. This will change as you practise and progress. You may start out with a modification of a pose, and in time, you will be able to do the final pose. After you become familiar with the postures, see if you can hold them for longer periods of time with a balance between ease and effort.

Seek the advice and knowledge of an experienced teacher if you are having problems with a pose. Go to classes with a knowledgeable teacher to enhance and deepen your home practice.

CHAPTER 9

Warm-Up Poses

Warm-up poses provide a safe transition into asana practice, isolating muscle groups and body parts, such as the shoulders, spine, hips, lower back and groin. You can use the warm-up sequence in this chapter in its entirety as a gentle practice, or try a few of the poses, depending upon your needs.

SUPTA VRKSASANA

Supta Vrksasana is the reclining mountain pose. Lie down with your feet together (SEE FIGURE 9-1). Stretch the heels and the balls of the feet forwards, as you fully stretch your legs away from the feet and ankles. Have your arms diagonally by your sides with the palms facing up.

FIGURE 9-1:
Supta
Vrksasana

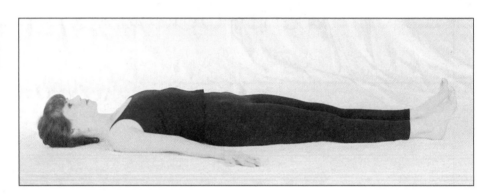

PAVANMUKTASANA

Pavanmuktasana is the wind-relieving pose. Lie down on your back with the knees bent and feet flat on the floor. Inhale fully. Exhale and draw the knees into the chest (SEE FIGURE 9-2). Hug the knees with the arms and stay for several breaths, savouring the stretching of the lower back muscles. Next, draw your chin toward your knees (SEE FIGURE 9-3), and hold for a few breaths.

FIGURE 9-2:
Drawing the
knees into the
chest in
Pavanmuktasana

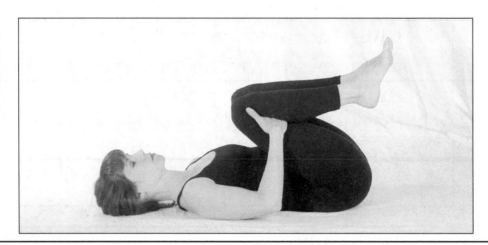

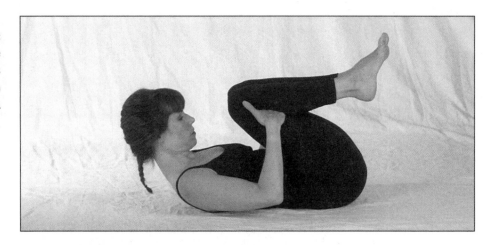

FIGURE 9-3:
Drawing the
chin towards
the knees in
Pavanmuktasana

MODIFIED SUPTA PADANGUSTHASANA

The Modified Supta Padangusthasana is the reclining-hand-on-the-big-toe pose. Still lying down, with your knees bent, extend your left leg onto the floor and stretch the foot forward. Clasp the hands behind the right knee (SEE FIGURE 9-4), and hold for several breaths.

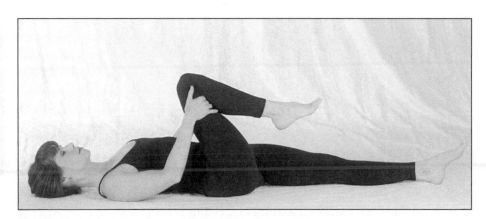

FIGURE 9-4:
Clasping the
hands behind
the knee in
Modified Supta
Padangusth-
asana

FIGURE 9-5:
Holding the
right leg
behind the
knee in
Modified Supta
Padangusth-
asana

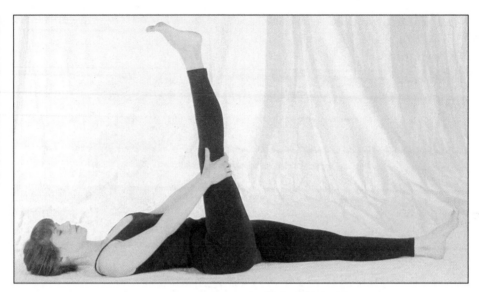

FIGURE 9-6:
Using a belt in
Modified Supta
Padangusth-
asana

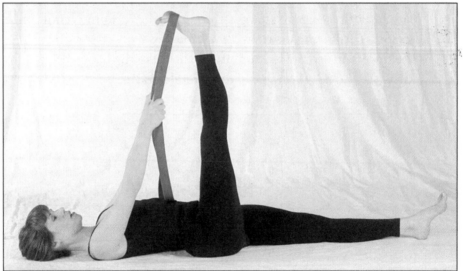

Then extend the right leg up, either holding behind the knee (SEE FIGURE 9-5) or holding onto a belt that is around the ball of the right foot (SEE FIGURE 9-6). Be in the pose, breathing smoothly, gently stretching the leg or keeping it slightly bent.

PAVANMUKTASANA WITH WIDE LEGS

Pavanmuktasana is also known as the child's pose; this pose is done with wide legs. Lying on your back, bend the knees into the chest and then bring the knees comfortably wide apart. Clasp the hands under the knees, holding onto the outside of the knee (SEE FIGURE 9-7). Stay in this position for several breaths. Then change the hand position, with the hands on the inside of the knee (SEE FIGURE 9-8).

FIGURE 9-7:
Holding the outside of the knees in Pavanmuktasana with Wide Legs

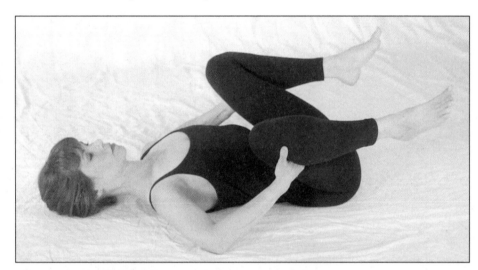

FIGURE 9-8:
Holding the inside of the knees in Pavanmuktasana with Wide Legs

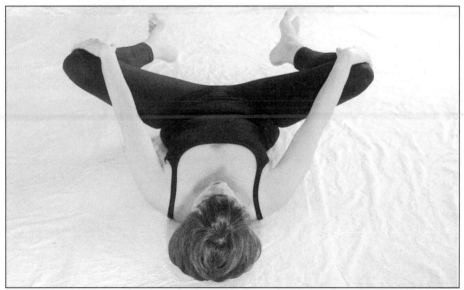

SUPINE SPINAL ROCK

Supine Spinal Rock is a great warm-up for the spine. Lying down, with hands clasped under your knees, tuck your chin into your chest and begin rolling up and down your spine, in a gentle, rocking motion (SEE FIGURES 9-9, 9-10 AND 9-11). Repeat several times.

FIGURE 9-9:
Rolling back in
the Supine
Spinal Rock

FIGURE 9-10:
Coming to
centre in
the Supine
Spinal Rock

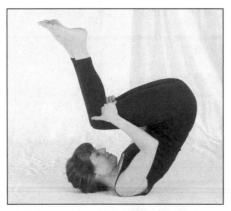

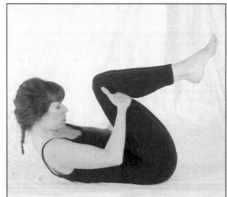

FIGURE 9-11:
Rolling
forward in
the Supine
Spinal Rock

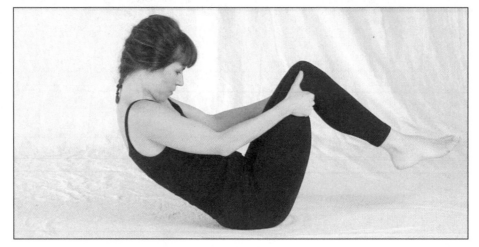

SUPTA BADDHA KONASANA

Supta Baddha Konasana is the cobbler's pose. Lie down, bend the knees out to the side and join the soles of the feet. Draw the feet in toward the pelvis, to where it is comfortable. Let the thighs release down to the floor (SEE FIGURE 9-12). Remain for several breaths.

FIGURE 9-12:
Supta Baddha Konasana

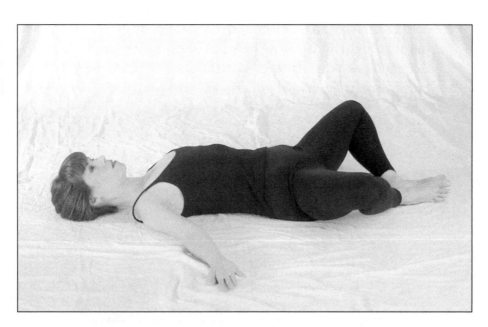

LEG CRADLE

The Leg Cradle is a great hip-opener. Lie down with your knees bent and feet flat on the floor. Bend your right leg out to the side and place the outside of your right ankle on the thigh close to the knee. Clasp your hands under the left knee by threading the right arm between the legs and wrapping the left arm around the outside of the left thigh to the knee (SEE FIGURE 9-13). Inhale and, on the exhalation, gently draw the left leg in toward the chest. As you do this, pull the buttock bones down towards the floor and press the left thigh into the clasped hands. Stay for several breaths and then change sides.

FIGURE 9-13:
Leg Cradle

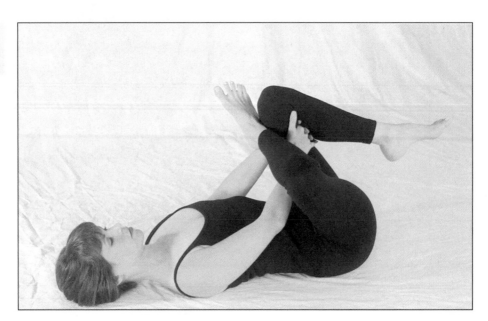

JATHARA PARIVARTANASANA

Jathara Parivartanasana is the stomach-turning pose. Lie down and bend the knees with the feet flat on the floor. Lift the feet away from the floor and bring the knees to the chest. Extend the arms horizontally on the floor. Stack the knees and ankles and let the knees come down to the floor on the left side at a 90° angle (SEE FIGURE 9-14). Gaze up at the ceiling. Feel the stomach and the ribs spiral toward the right. Maintain the length of the spine upon inhalation, twist on the exhalation and roll the right shoulder down toward the floor (without forcing). Stay in the pose for several breaths, deepening the twist. Then bring the knees back to the centre and repeat on the other side.

FIGURE 9-14:
Jathara
Parivartan-
asana

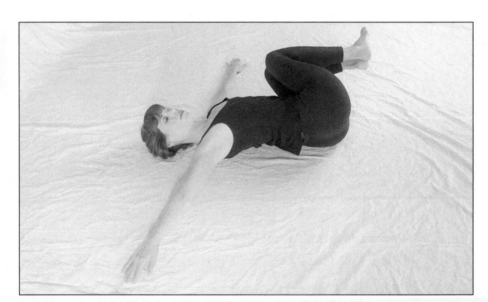

SPHINX POSE

Lie on your front with legs extended behind you. Prop yourself up on your forearms. Your forearms will be parallel to each other, with the elbows close to the waist and in line with the wrists and shoulders (SEE FIGURE 9-15). Press the forearms and the palms down, and observe how this grounding action lifts the chest and elongates the sides of the body. Maintaining this action, pull the elbows back on the floor without actually moving them. Feel the muscles of the upper back draw in to the back and hug the shoulder blades. Enhance this by lifting the sternum forward and up. Enjoy the openness and broadness of the chest. Stay for several breaths and then release and rest.

FIGURE 9-15:
Sphinx Pose

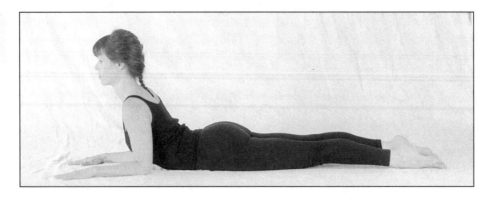

SALABHASANA SINGLE LEG LIFT

Salabhasana is the locust pose. Lie on your front and rest your head on your forearms. Extend the legs behind you. Inhale and lift the left leg slightly off the floor (SEE FIGURE 9-16). As you exhale, stretch the leg from the hip to the toes, then release the leg down to the floor and repeat on the other side. This pose can be repeated two to three times.

FIGURE 9-16:
Salabhasana
Single Leg Lift

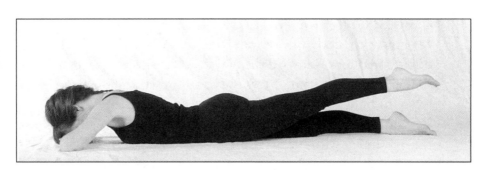

MODIFIED ARDHA BHEKASANA

Ardha Bhekasana is the half-frog pose. Lying on your front, bend the left leg and hold onto the left outer ankle with the left hand (SEE FIGURE 9-17). With each exhalation, soften into the pose, allowing the front of the thigh to open and the hamstring to contract. Do not practise this pose if you suffer from knee pain.

FIGURE 9-17:
Modified Ardha
Bhekasana

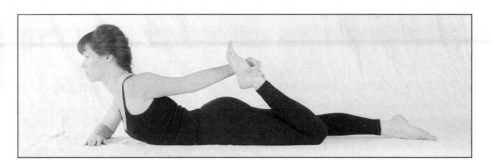

CAT POSE

This pose warms up the spine beautifully, creating suppleness and stretching the back muscles. Start on all fours, with wrists under shoulders and knees under hips. Look forward and lengthen into the crown of the head and into the coccyx. Slightly tip the coccyx up (SEE FIGURE 9-18). Inhale the breath. Press the inner thighs away from each other, hugging the bone. Exhale and round the spine by curling the chin into the chest and lifting each vertebra up toward the ceiling (SEE FIGURE 9-19). Draw the coccyx in between the legs toward the pubis bone. The pubis bones moves toward the navel, and the navel recedes and presses up to the front of the spine. Press the hands down and push the hands away from the body as you round the back. Repeat the lengthening on the inhalation and rounding on the exhalation nine more times, coordinating the movement with the breath.

FIGURE 9-18:
The beginning position of the Cat Pose

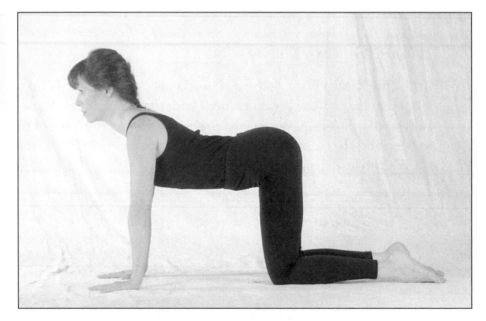

FIGURE 9-19:
The ending
position of the
Cat Pose

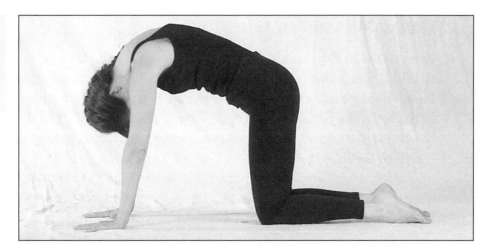

BALASANA

Balasana is the child's pose. Start on the hands and knees, with the hands under the shoulders and the knees under the hips. Inhale, and on the exhalation draw your buttocks back to rest on your heels. Press the hands on the floor, extending into the fingertips and stretching back through the sides of the body to the hips (SEE FIGURE 9-20). Let the forehead rest on the floor. While in the pose, inhale and feel the expansion of the waist and lower back. Exhale and observe the contraction of the ribs and lungs and the softening of the body as the breath leaves the body. Stay for several breaths and then come back up and release the pose.

For enhanced lengthening of the spine, practice balasana by walking the hands to the right for several breaths and then to the left. This stretch isolates the action on one side of the body at a time.

FIGURE 9-20:
Balasana

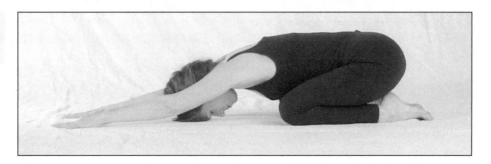

PARVATASANA IN VAJRASANA

Parvatasana in Vajrasana is the thunderbolt pose. Sit in Dandasana (refer to p 132) then come into a kneeling position with the spine upright and long. The shins and the front of the feet are on the floor. Plant the buttocks on the heels. Lift and open the top chest and lengthen through the crown of the head. Soften the eyes, throat, diaphragm and stomach. Interlock the fingers with arms in front of you. Inhale and raise the arms up over the head. Press the upper arms in toward the head and stretch up through the forearms. Spread and broaden the palms (SEE FIGURES 9-21 AND 9-22). Stay for several breaths, then exhale and release the interlock. Change the interlock and repeat the pose.

FIGURE 9-21:
Parvatasana in
Vajrasana: side
view

FIGURE 9-22:
Parvatasana in
Vajrasana: front
view

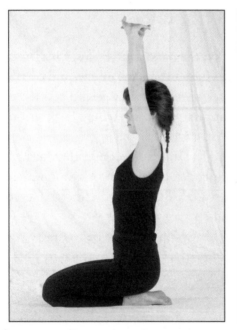
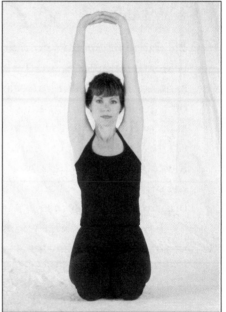

GOMUKHASANA ARMS WHILE SITTING IN VAJRASANA

Gomukhasana is the cow's head pose; Vajrasana is the thunderbolt pose. Extend the right arm up. Wrap the left arm behind the body. Bend the elbows and see if you can clasp the fingers of each hand together on the back, between the shoulders (SEE FIGURE 9-23). If not, use a strap or belt (SEE FIGURE 9-24). Stretch the elbows away from each other and pull the fingers as if trying to draw them apart. Bring the right arm up and back, with the inner arm next to the right ear. Draw the left shoulder back to bring the shoulder blade into the body. Expand the ribcage with the breath, and lengthen the sides of the body equally. Lift and broaden the collarbones. Stay for several breaths. Note the quality of your breathing: breath that is easy indicates balance, while erratic breathing or holding the breath indicates over-striving. Repeat on the other side.

FIGURE 9-23:
Gomukhasana
Arms While
Sitting in
Vajrasana

FIGURE 9-24:
Gomukhasana
Arms While
Sitting in
Vajrasana, using
a strap

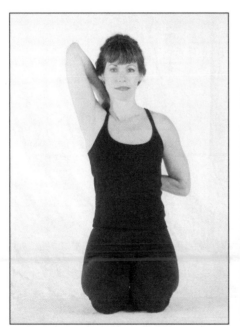
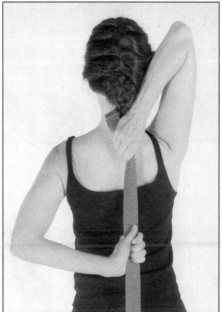

GARUDASANA ARMS IN VAJRASANA
WITH TOES TUCKED UNDER

Garudasana is the eagle pose; Vajrasana is the thunderbolt pose. Tuck in
your toes. Extend the arms horizontally out to the sides. Inhale the breath.
Exhale deeply and quickly intertwine the arms, elbow over elbow, wrist,
over wrist and palms together (SEE FIGURE 9-25). Inhale and feel the breath fill
the area between the shoulder blades. Exhale and soften the shoulder area.
Stretch the muscles of the back body. Stay for several breaths. Release and
repeat by changing the arm that crosses over on top of the other arm.

FIGURE 9-25:
Garudasana
Arms in
Vajrasana with
Toes Tucked
Under

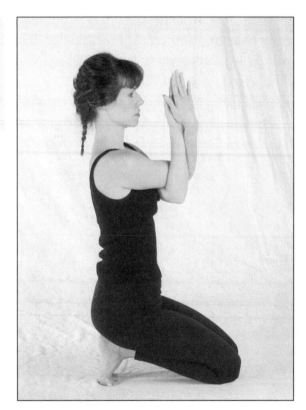

SUKHASANA SIDE STRETCH

Sukhasana is an easy pose. Sit cross-legged with your arms by your sides. The left palm is on the floor by the outside of the left hip. Stretch the right arm out to the side with the palm facing up. Lengthen all the way from the centre of the body to the fingertips. Inhale and stretch the right arm up. Press the buttock bones down and stretch up through the right side of the body to the fingertips. Exhale and bend laterally to the left. Stretch the right arm over the head, in line with the right ear (SEE FIGURE 9-26). With every inhalation, re-establish the grounding of the buttocks bones, and with every exhalation deepen the stretch. Release the right arm down to the side. Repeat on the other side.

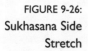

FIGURE 9-26:
Sukhasana Side
Stretch

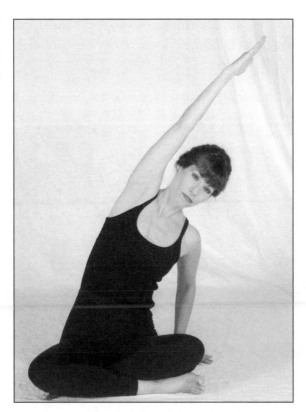

ARDHA MANDALASANA

Ardha Mandalasana is the lunge pose. Come onto all fours. Look forward, bend the left leg, swing it forward and plant the left foot between the hands. Spread the toes and the balls of the feet, and lift the arches. The left shin is perpendicular to the floor, with the knee over the heel. Extend the right leg from the hip to the heel with the toes tucked under (SEE FIGURE 9-27). Lift the back thigh away from the floor slightly, to ensure that the thighbone is feeding into the socket, rather than hanging out of the socket (hanging from the hip joint is detrimental to the health of the joint and its surrounding ligaments and tendons). Ground the left foot and toes of the right foot. Maintain the extension of the spine from the coccyx to the crown of the head. Press the fingertips into the floor as you stretch the arms up into the shoulder sockets to support the upper body. Hold the pose for several breaths. Then release back onto all fours. Repeat on the left side.

FIGURE 9-27:
Ardha
Mandalasana

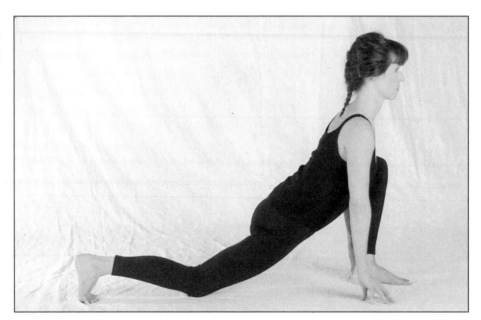

ARDHA UTTANASANA ON CHAIR

Ardha Uttanasana is the half-standing forward bend. Place the hands on a chair seat and hold onto the sides of the chair seat without tension. As the hands ground into the chair, the arms stretch back into the shoulder sockets. The elbows firm and straighten (SEE FIGURE 9-28). Continue lengthening from the shoulders to the buttock bones. Press the shoulder blades into the back. The body is parallel to the floor, with the head between the arms. If the head is either lower or higher than the arms, the neck and head will be out of line with the rest of the spine. The crown of the head stretches forward as the coccyx lengthens back. The heels are directly under the hips and the feet are hip width (or wider) apart (depending upon the comfort of your hamstrings – tight hamstrings require a wider leg stance). The body is parallel to the floor.

Make sure that you are not pressing the shoulders or front ribs down in an effort to open the body. You want a long line of stretch from the fingertips to the buttock bones and from the buttock bones to the heels.

Broaden the lower back by spreading the buttock bones away from each other, letting the inner thighs hug the thigh bones (away from each other). Pull the hips and the tops of the thighs back toward the middle of the room to create even more length in the spine. Feel the terrific space and length in the torso and the back of the legs. Stay for a few breaths and enjoy the space you have created in your body.

FIGURE 9-28:
Ardha
Uttanasana
on Chair

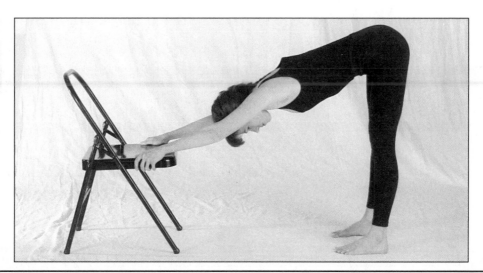

ELBOWS ON THE CHAIR

Kneel in front of the chair. Place the tips of your elbows on the front edge of the chair. Press the palms and fingers together into prayer position. Have the head between the arms (SEE FIGURE 9-29). Stretch from the elbows to the hips and lengthen your spine from the crown of the head to the coccyx. The body is parallel to the floor.

FIGURE 9-29:
Elbows on
the Chair

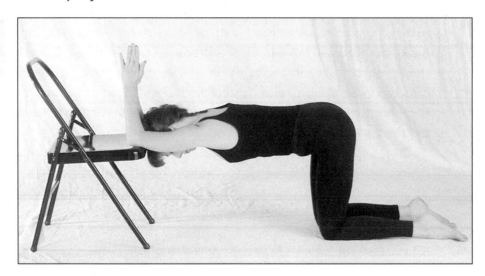

ADHO MUKHA SVANASANA

Adho Mukha Svanasana is the downward-facing dog pose. Begin on your hands and knees (SEE FIGURE 9-30). Inhale your breath and lift the hips high (SEE FIGURE 9-31). Press down through the hands and stretch up through the arms to the buttock bones. Ground the feet as you stretch from the heels to the buttocks, lengthening the legs (SEE FIGURE 9-32).

FIGURE 9-30:
Beginning
Adho Mukha
Svanasana on
hands and
knees

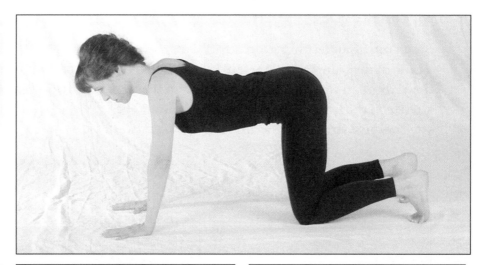

FIGURE 9-31:
Lifting
the hips

FIGURE 9-32:
Lengthening
the legs

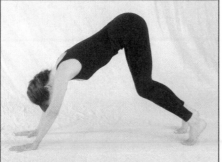
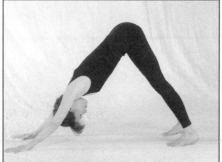

UTKATASANA

Utkatasana is the chair pose. Stand with the feet hip-width apart. Bend the hips, knees and ankles as if you were about to sit down. Bring the weight back into the heels. Extend the arms out to the sides, palms facing up. Inhale and stretch the arms up (SEE FIGURE 9-33).

STANDING SIDE STRETCH

Stand with your feet hip-width apart. Extend your right arm out to the side with the palm facing up. Inhale and stretch the right arm up. Press down through your feet as you stretch into the right fingertips. Feel the stretch on the right side of the body. Exhale and bend to the left side as you continue stretching the arm over the head (SEE FIGURE 9-34).

FIGURE 9-33:
Utkatasana

FIGURE 9-34:
Standing
Side Stretch

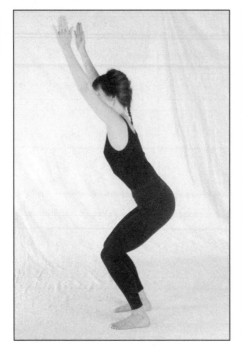

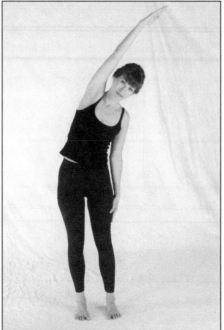

TADASANA WITH HANDS CLASPED BEHIND THE BACK

Tadasana is the mountain pose (refer to p104). Stand with your feet hip-width apart and clasp your hands behind you. Inhale and, as you exhale, gently pull the arms away from the body. Lift the sternum and observe the opening and expansion of the chest. Stay for several breaths. Then bend forward from the hips, letting the arms come down towards the head (SEE FIGURE 9-35). Inhale and slowly come up as you press the feet down. Change the clasp of the hands and repeat.

FIGURE 9-35:
Tadasana with
Hands Clasped
Behind
the Back

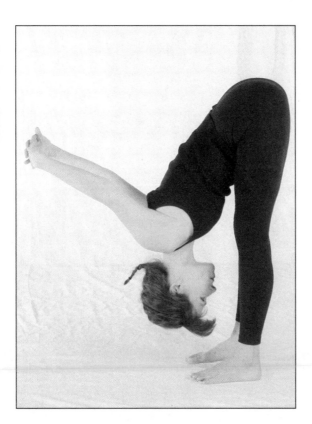

CHAPTER 10
Standing Poses

S tanding poses help develop correct alignment from the feet up. They open the hips, stretch the legs fully, strengthen the back and increase range of movement. Digestion, elimination and circulation are improved. Arms and legs stretch completely while fully supporting the torso. Standing postures are strenuous and contribute to weight loss.

TADASANA

Tadasana, the mountain pose, is the basic standing pose. Like a mountain, you want a broad, stable base from which to extend to the sky. Tadasana teaches you how to stand properly. You learn how to balance, centre, ground and extend.

Start by placing your feet together, joining the big toes and inner ankles, if possible. Otherwise, stand so the ankles, knees and hips are lined up, one over the other. When viewed from one side, the ear, shoulder, hip, knee and ankle should form a straight, vertical line, with your arms by your sides (SEE FIGURE 10-1).

FIGURE 10-1:
Tadasana

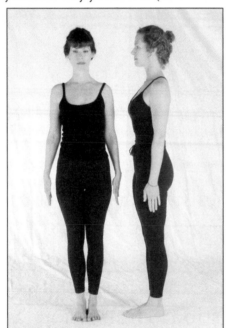

Create your yoga feet by spreading the toes and balls of the feet, pressing into the big and little toe mounds and the centre of the heel. Bring the weight a little more into the heels. Lift your arches as you ground the feet. Enhance this action by lengthening your leg muscles all the way up to your hips. Lift the top of the kneecaps up by contracting the quadricep muscle. Firm the muscles of the thigh to the bone.

Now you have created a strong and stable base from which the torso will be able to extend. This is like creating the mantle for the mountain to rise out of. Place your hands on your hips and extend the sides of the body from your hips to your armpits. This action creates length and space in the spine.

Bring your arms back to your sides without losing the lift of the spine, lengthen up through the crown of your head. Try to balance your head over the pelvis. Make sure the shoulders are relaxed and are not riding up to the ears. Press your shoulder blades into your back. Lift the top of your chest and broaden the collarbones. Breathe fully, balancing ease with effort. Open the body to receive the breath, remaining aware of how it feels to be in alignment. Be the observer and the observed, the seer and the seen.

Tadasana can be done with the back to the wall for alignment. The tactile feedback from the back on the wall will aid in the sense of lengthening the torso. Tadasana can also be performed lying down, with the feet flush against the wall. This is an excellent way to feel the two-way action of the feet pressing, spreading and lengthening in one direction, while the legs grow long in the opposite direction. The muscle action of the legs hugging the bone is also more pronounced when lying down, because the floor provides feedback, and there is no need to balance on the feet, as when standing.

The benefits of Tadasana include the following:

· It teaches you how to stand correctly with proper alignment.
· It develops agility.
· It corrects minor misalignments of legs.
· It strengthens ankles.
· It relieves backache and neck strain.
· It opens the chest.

The next time you find yourself waiting in a queue at the supermarket, use the time as an opportunity to practise yoga. Stand in Tadasana. Ground your feet, fully stretch your legs and lengthen your spine from the coccyx to the crown of the head. Breathe through your nostrils and expand and lift the chest.

UTTHITA HASTA PADANGUSTHASANA I

Utthita Hasta Padangusthasana I is the extended-hand-on-the-foot posture. Stand in Tadasana, facing a chair. Transfer the weight onto the left leg and foot. Lift the right leg up and place the back of the right heel on the chair. Determine whether your hamstring flexibility allows you to place your foot on the chair seat (SEE FIGURE 10-2) or on the top of the chair back (SEE FIGURE 10-3). Place a belt around the ball of the right foot and hold the straps with each hand. Observe that the outer left hip and ankle are in line. Stretch both legs fully as you lengthen into both active yoga feet. Press down into the right heel as you lengthen up through the back of the leg and the spine to the crown of the head.

FIGURE 10-2:
Utthita Hasta Padangusth-asana I with foot on chair seat

FIGURE 10-3:
Utthita Hasta Padangusth-asana I with foot on chair back

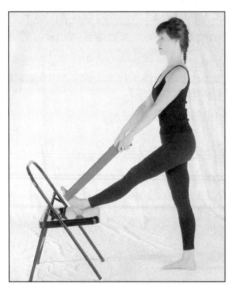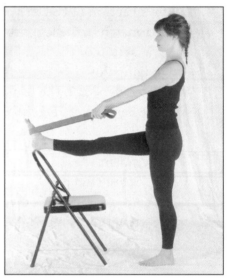

Try to keep both legs straight by the equal and opposite reactions of pressing into the feet, lifting the arches and fully stretching up through the legs, lifting the kneecaps, contracting the quadriceps muscles and hugging the thigh muscles to the bone. Contract the quadriceps faster than you lengthen the back of the knee. Do not lock the knees, because this will cause hyperextension. Stretch the whole body up, lifting the ribs and elongating both sides of the body. Try to keep the buttocks level with each other, so one hip is not higher than the other. Stay in the pose for a few breaths. Breathe softly and fully, receiving the breath and balancing ease and effort. On the exhalation, bring the arms and leg down. Then repeat on the other side.

Utthita Hasta Padangusthasana I strengthens and tones the legs, stretches the hamstrings and develops balance and poise.

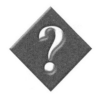

What is Ayurveda?

Ayurveda and yoga are two closely intertwined disciplines from ancient India. *Ayurveda* means 'knowledge of life'. According to Ayurveda, everything is made up of three different energies called *doshas*. The three doshas are *vatta, pitta* and *kapha*. Everyone has their own unique combination of the doshas, which is determined at conception.

UTTHITA TRIKONASANA

Utthita Trikonasana is the extended triangle pose. Begin by standing in Tadasana. Walk your feet 1.2–1.3m (4ft–4ft 6in) apart and actively stretch your arms, all the way from the heart to the fingertips. Feel the opening of the chest and the upper ribs as a result of the active stretch of the arms. Turn your left foot in 15° and revolve your right leg out. The right foot is at a 110° to 120° angle to the left foot, and the right and left heels are in line with each other. The right leg is the front leg and the left leg is the back leg. Plant and spread your active yoga feet and lift the inner and outer arches up. Inhale, lengthening up through the legs and stretching them fully. Maintain the lifting of the kneecaps by contracting the quadriceps. Exhale. Elongate the sides of the body as you inhale and expand your lungs and lift the ribs. Exhale and extend laterally over your right leg, bending from the hip. Remember, it is not about how far you go down to the side, it's about being strong, extended and balanced, while moving directly to the side over the right leg. This helps keep the pose in your legs so the spine can maintain its length and freedom.

Place the right fingertips lightly on the right shin. Keep extending through both arms and equally through both sides of the body. Have the head in line with the spine and lengthen from the crown of the head to the coccyx. Look straight ahead. Try to keep the back of the body in one plane. Frequently, the upper body is leaning forward of the lower body.

Find the balance between ease and effort. Is your breath ragged or held, indicating over-effort, or is it smooth and even, indicating ease?

Maintain the pose for several breaths. See if you can continue elongating the body and opening the chest with every inhalation. Breathe normally. Inhale and come up out of the pose by grounding the feet and stretching up and back into your left hand. Release the arms to your sides, bring the feet to parallel, and repeat on the other side.

FIGURE 10-4:
Utthita
Trikonasana
using a chair

FIGURE 10-5:
Utthita
Trikonasana
using a block

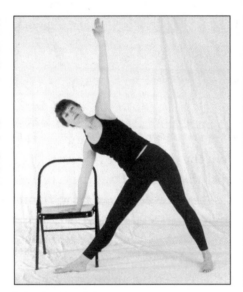

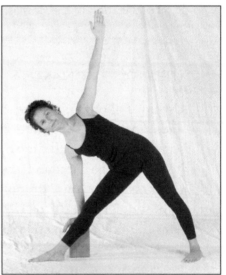

FIGURE 10-6:
Utthita
Trikonasana:
final pose

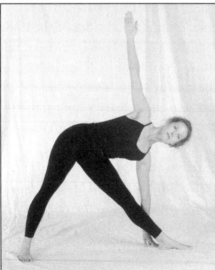

As a modification of this pose, start by standing with legs wide apart. Have a chair behind you, by the right ankle. Come into the pose, as described earlier, and place your right hand on the chair. Press the right hand down as you stretch up through the right arm to the left fingertips (SEE FIGURE 10-4). Or use a block behind the front ankle to place the hand on (SEE FIGURE 10-5). This allows for greater lengthening of the spine. Trikonasana can also be done against the wall for support and alignment (SEE FIGURE 10-6). The outer heel of the back leg can be against the wall for stability and balance. This way Trikonasana teaches the strong lengthening and grounding action of the back leg and foot.

The benefits of Trikonasana include the following:

· It strengthens and balances the muscles of the legs, hips and spine.
· It lengthens the back and abdominal muscles, providing space for the internal organs and length for the spine.
· It relieves back pain.
· It teaches sense of direction and lateral extension.
· It gives the intercostal muscles between the ribs a powerful stretch, allowing for greater lung capacity and fuller, deeper breathing.
· It expands the chest.

Standing poses can be done with the back against the wall for support and correct alignment. The wall is a great (silent) teacher, showing you where you really are in space. These poses are also beneficial for those with back problems, cardiac problems or nervous system disorders, and for pregnant women and those recovering from an illness or surgery, provided they have checked with their doctor.

PARIVRITTA TRIKONASANA

Parivritta Trikonasana, the revolved triangle pose, is the counterpose to Utthita Trikonasana. It is a challenging posture, containing a forward bend, a balance and a twist.

Stand in Tadasana and jump or walk the legs wide apart. Inhale and raise and extend the arms actively out to the sides. Turn the left foot in 45° to 60° and revolve the right leg out so the foot is at 90°. On an exhalation, turn the body completely to face the right leg. Revolve the back (left) leg so the front of the thigh faces forward. Turn toward the right as you extend the torso, and place your left hand on the floor by the outside of the right foot. Place the right palm on the lower back. Continue revolving the torso around the axis of the spine as you extend from the crown of the head to the coccyx. Then extend the right arm up, stretching into the fingertips (SEE FIGURE 10-7).

FIGURE 10-7:
Parivritta
Trikonasana

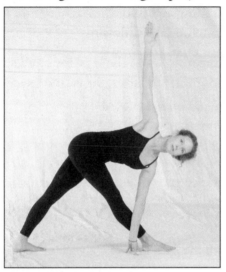

To help with balance, press strongly into your active yoga feet and draw the hips and upper thighs back behind you to balance the forward movement of your body. Draw the kneecap, quadricep and hamstring muscles firmly up the leg.

Inhale the breath, hug the muscles to the bone and come up out of the pose with strong legs, taking care not to lose the grounding of the feet as you do this. Turn the feet back to parallel and the body back to the centre. Release the arms down to the sides. Pause and then repeat on the other side.

You can practise this pose by placing a chair to your right, with the chair seat turned to face your right side. Stand with the legs wide apart and turn the back foot in more than 45°. Revolve the front leg out, so the foot is under the chair seat. Come into Parivritta Trikonasana, and place the right hand on the chair seat and the left palm on the small of the back as you revolve your body toward the right (SEE FIGURE 10-8). Or you can use a block by the inside of the front shin to place the hand on (SEE FIGURE 10-9). As you become more familiar and at ease with the pose, place the block by the outside of the shin and cross the hand over the leg onto the block. As another alternative, you can position the back outer heel against the wall for stability and support. This will help with balance and ease. Practise the pose against the wall. Have the front leg side against the wall. As you come forward and turn toward the wall, place both hands, with arms extended, on the wall. Continue lengthening and revolving in the pose with the support of the wall.

FIGURE 10-8:
Parivritta
Trikonasana,
using a chair

FIGURE 10-9:
Parivritta
Trikonasana,
using a block

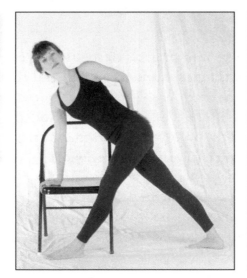
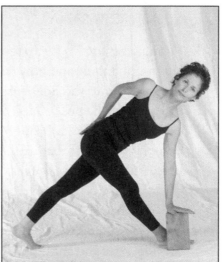

The benefits of Parivritta Trikonasana include the following:

- It develops balance and coordination.
- It provides a long, diagonal stretch of the torso muscles from shoulder to hip and massages the body organs.
- It expands the chest.
- It strongly works the legs.
- It strengthens the hip muscles.
- It eases back pain.
- It reduces fat around the waist and hips.
- It decreases sciatic pain.
- It reduces arthritic pain.

Jumping in and out of yoga poses helps develop agility. However, if you have back or knee problems, jumping in and out of poses is not recommended. Walking in and out of the poses works well, too.

VIRABHADRASANA I

Virabhadrasana I is a warrior pose. Warrior poses create strength of body and mind. Inhale and jump or walk the feet wide apart. Lift and extend the arms out to the sides from the centre of the body to the fingertips throughout the pose. Open and lift the chest as you inhale. Keep the chest expanded and lifted throughout the pose (without protruding the front ribs). Turn the left foot in 15° and revolve the right leg out 90°, heel in line with heel. Press the feet firmly down.

Inhale the breath and create extension in the body from the feet up to the fingertips. Exhale fully and bend the right leg to a 90° angle, with the knee over the ankle. The entire leg bends to achieve this, not just the knee. The hip, knee and ankle bend. The right thigh descends down toward the floor. (If you cannot get into a 90° angle, don't worry, just do the best you can without force or strain). As the right leg bends, the left leg remains long. The left foot actively grounds, especially on the outer edge of the foot. The left kneecap lifts up as the quadricep muscle contracts.

There is a dynamic interplay and balance between the action of the legs. As much as the right leg bends, that's how much the left leg straightens through extension and grounding. Become aware of this duality, and try to maintain a balance between the two actions.

The arms continue to extend out from the centre line of the body with the shoulder blades pressing into the back, supporting the upper body (SEE FIGURE 10-10). The body remains centred between the legs. To achieve this, stretch even more into the left arm and fingertips, so the body remains upright.

FIGURE 10-10:
Virabhadr-
asana I

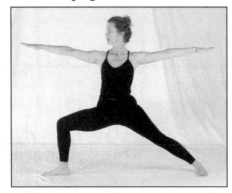

The tendency is for the body to lean towards the bent leg. This causes undue strain to the right knee. Imagine that someone is holding onto your left hand and pulling you out of the pose.

Maintain the length and extension of the torso. Lift the ribcage away from the hips, and bring the hips down. Feel the space created in the abdomen and the lower back. Gaze toward your right hand and remain for several breaths. To come out of the pose, look forwards, press down into your right foot and lift the kneecap and quadricep up to lengthen the right leg, then turn the feet parallel. Repeat on the other side.

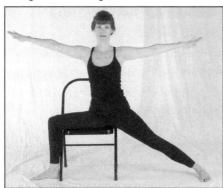

FIGURE 10-11: Virabhad-rasana I, using a chair

You can also practise this pose while sitting on a chair. Bend the right leg out to the side and slide the thigh to the left, so the right thigh is completely supported on the chair. The left leg is now off the chair. Extend the left leg out to the side, grounding and spreading the foot and lifting the arches. Lift through the sides of the body as you extend the arms out to the sides (SEE FIGURE 10-11). Repeat on the other side. If you prefer, you can stand with your back to the wall for support and alignment. Place the back outer heel against wall for stability and support.

The benefits of Virabhadrasana II include the following:

· It teaches coordination of movement and breath, as well as correct alignment.
· It increases strength in the abdominal, back, buttock and leg muscles, which contribute to the support of the spine.
· It tones the abdomen.
· The legs, pelvic girdle and buttocks stretch and open.

tips

The active extending of the arms and legs out of the body must be balanced by a drawing of muscle action in from the periphery to the core. Extension by itself will not create space in the body or promote health of the joints or the tendons and ligaments supporting them.

UTTHITA PARSVAKONASANA

In the Utthita Parsvakonasana posture (the extended side-angle pose), there is a long diagonal stretch on the upper side of the body, all the way from the foot to the fingertips. Start in Tadasana and jump or walk the legs wide apart to a comfortable distance (even wider than Trikonasana). Extend the arms out to the sides. Turn the left foot in 15°, and revolve the right leg out. Heel is in line with heel. Ground the feet, spread the toes and lift the arches. Keeping the feet active, firm the muscles to the bone throughout the posture to keep the energy flowing, to support the knees and to maintain a stable base of the legs and feet.

Inhale through the nostrils, infusing the body with the breath as if you were smelling a pleasing fragrance, and lengthen up through the legs and the sides of the body. This will lift and expand the chest. Exhale fully as you bend the right leg (at the hip, knee and ankle), with the knee in line with the heel. The leg will form a 90° angle. Bend the torso from the hips directly to the side over the right leg, and bring the right hand behind the right foot, fingertips touching the ground. Turn the left arm up from the shoulder. Inhale and extend the left arm up and over the head (SEE FIGURE 10-12). This external rotation of the left arm flattens the shoulder blade on the back and opens the chest.

FIGURE 10-12:
Utthita
Parsvak-
onasana

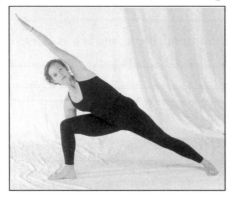

As you firm the outer edge of the left foot down, lengthen up the left side of the body into the fingertips. Stretch into the fingertips and elongate both sides of the body evenly. Look straight ahead, with the chest facing forward, keep the head in line with the spine, and observe the marvellous diagonal stretch you have created on the left side of the body. Stretch into the crown of the head and into the coccyx. Continue breathing naturally and smoothly.

Elongate the right side from the hip to the armpit. Keep the shoulder blades on the back. Feel the opening and stretching of the pelvis. Stay in the pose for a few breaths. Enjoy this strong, dynamic stretch, moving past all limitations. Keep reaching. Come up out of the pose pressing into the right foot, lengthening the right leg and reaching out the left arm. Turn the feet back to parallel, and then repeat on the other side.

You can practise the pose with the forearm on the thigh or on a chair (behind you), instead of bringing the hand to the floor behind the foot (SEE FIGURE 10-13). This will ensure proper alignment until you are ready to progress to the classic pose. You can also place the back hand on a block (SEE FIGURE 10-14), or stand with the back against the wall for support and alignment. Place the back outer heel against the wall for support and grounding.

FIGURE 10-13:
Utthita
Parsvak-
onasana, using
a chair

FIGURE 10-14:
Utthita
Parsvak-
onasana, using
a block

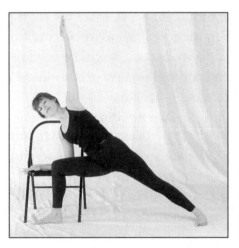
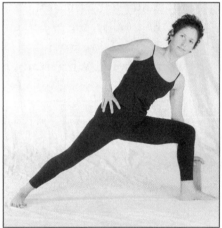

The benefits of Utthita Parsvakonasana include the following:

· It strengthens the muscles of the legs and the back.
· It opens the shoulders, hips and groin.
· It tones the oblique abdominal muscles.
· It tones the ankles and knees.
· It reduces body fat around the waist and hips.
· It expands the chest.
· It reduces sciatic and arthritic pain.
· It improves digestion.

PARIVRITTA PARSVAKONASANA

Parivritta Parsvakonasana, the reverse extended side-angle pose, adds a twist and the element of balance to Utthita Parsvakonasana. Begin by standing in Tadasana. Walk or jump the feet wide apart. Extend the arms from the heart to the fingertips. Turn the left foot way in, 45° to 60°. Turn the right leg out to 90°. Inhale the breath, and on the exhalation turn to face the front leg. Inhale and extend up from the grounding of the feet into the fingertips. Exhale completely and bend the front leg. Bend forward from the hips and turn your whole body to face your right leg.

Press the left fingertips down on the floor by the outside of the right foot and extend the arm into the shoulder socket. Place the right palm on the small of the back. Lengthen the spine as you inhale and further revolve the body around the spine as you exhale. Keep the head in line with the spine. When ready, extend the arm up and over the head (SEE FIGURE 10-15). Otherwise, leave the palm on the small of the back.

FIGURE 10-15:
Parivritta
Parsvakon-
asana

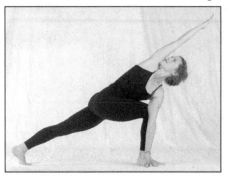

Do not force or strain in the twist. Relax the effort slightly and then see if you can twist a little more. Breathe.

Carefully come out of the twist as you exhale. Plant the feet firmly until fully firm, and stretch the legs as you bring the body upright. Bring the feet to parallel, centre the body and release the arms . Repeat on the other side.

You can also practise this pose by placing the left forearm on a chair seat behind you and the right palm on the small of the back (SEE FIGURE 10-16). Or place a block on the inside of the right foot to support the right hand (SEE FIGURE 10-17). After practising the pose for a while, put the block on the outside of the foot. This will increase the intensity and twist in the posture. Be aware if this is too much for you, and, if so go back and continue with the basic pose.

FIGURE 10-16:
Modified
Parivritta
Parsvakon-
asana, using a
chair

FIGURE 10-17:
With hand
on block

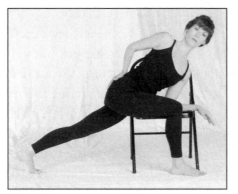
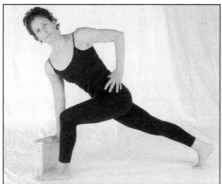

The benefits of Parivritta Parsvakonasana include the following:

- It helps with digestion and elimination as the intense twisting action of the pose contracts and massages the abdominal organs.
- It gives a powerful diagonal stretch to the back muscles.
- It loosens the hips and shoulders.
- It trims the waist and abdomen.
- It relieves sciatic pain.
- It reduces arthritic discomfort.

VIRABHADRASANA II

Virabhadrasana II, a warrior pose, is a vigorous posture that provides a tremendous stretch to the torso, spine and back leg. Begin by standing in Tadasana. Jump or walk the legs 1.2m (4ft) apart. Extend the arms out to the sides, palms facing up. Stretch into the fingertips and feel the opening of the chest and ribs. Inhale and lift the arms up over the head (SEE FIGURE 10-18, p120).

Connect the stretch of the side ribs with the lifting of the arms. Keep the palms facing each other, lengthen the arms and firm the elbows. If the elbows bend, bring the arms wider apart, in the shape of a **V**. By straightening the elbows, you will enhance the lifting of the side ribs and the extension of the spine.

FIGURE 10-18:
Virabhadr-
asana Ii

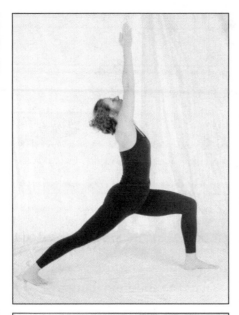

FIGURE 10-19:
Virabhadr-
asana Ii,
with thigh
on chair

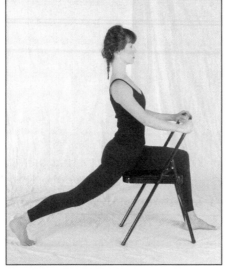

Turn the left foot in (45° to 60°) and revolve the left leg out. On an exhalation, turn your body to face the left (front) leg. Ground through the feet, lift the arches and extend all the way from the feet to the legs, the side body and the fingertips. Relax the top of the shoulders away from the ears to maintain the length of the neck and to release shoulder tension. Keep the eyes, face and throat soft.

Inhale the breath for extension, and as you exhale, bend the left leg (knee over ankle) and lengthen the right leg, pressing the top of the right thigh back. Don't worry if the right heel comes slightly off the floor. Lengthen the right leg from the hip to the heel. Bend the left leg, with the intention of creating a right angle. Continue to stretch from the side ribs into the fingertips to maintain lift and extension in the body. Stay for a few breaths. Observe your breath. Is it even and smooth, indicating stability and ease? Is it ragged, or are you holding the breath due to over-exertion?

Come out of the pose by pressing the feet firmly into the floor, carefully lengthening the front leg, turning the feet to parallel, facing the centre, bringing the arms down and jumping the feet back to Tadasana. Repeat on the other side.

You can also practise this pose using a chair (SEE FIGURE 10-19). Place the thigh of the front leg on the chair seat and sit down on that side. Keep the thigh completely supported. Bend the leg so the foot is flat on the floor. Hold onto the top of the chair back with the hands. Extend the back leg behind you, lengthening the groin back, tucking the toes under and stretching into the back heel. Ground the front foot. Lift and lengthen the sides of the body from the hips to the armpits. Change sides. For stability, you can place the outer heel of the back leg against a wall.

The benefits of Virabhadrasana II include the following:

· It develops balance and coordination.
· It develops strength in the legs.
· It opens the groin.
· It stretches and tones the abdomen.
· It increases stamina.
· It improves digestion.
· It relieves backache.
· It strengthens the bladder.
· It strengthens the the back muscles.
· It relieves menstrual pain and decreases heavy periods when practised before and after (not during) menstruation.

This posture is not recommended for those people with high blood pressure or cardiac disorders, unless it is practiced with the hands on the hips.

ARDHA CHANDRASANA

Ardha Chandrasana is the half-moon pose. To begin, come into Utthika Trikonasana. Walk your feet wide apart. Raise and extend the arms out to the sides. Turn the right foot in 15° and revolve the left leg out. Inhale from the legs and lift the ribs, and on the exhalation come into Trikonasana (SEE FIGURE 10-20, overleaf). Pause for a moment and enjoy the pose. Look forwards throughout the pose, instead of turning the head to look down. Place your right hand on your hip and keep it there.

FIGURE 10-20:
Going into
Ardha
Chandrasana
(final
Trikonasana
pose)

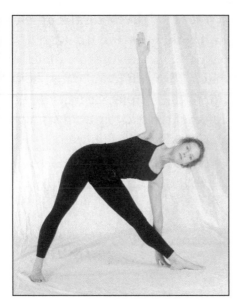

As you reach out with your left hand, bend the left leg to a right angle and place the fingertips of the left hand firmly on the floor, several inches in front of the left toes. Simultaneously walk the back leg towards the front. Draw your arm up into the shoulder socket from the cupping action of your fingertips (SEE FIGURE 10-21). If your fingers do not reach the floor, use a block to bring the floor to you.

Press into the left foot, stretch the leg fully and draw the standing leg muscles up to the hip socket. At the same time, lift the right leg up parallel to the floor (SEE FIGURE 10-22). Pull up the standing leg kneecap. Extend through the right heel and balls of the foot to maintain energy and firmness in the leg.

FIGURE 10-21:
Going into
Ardha
Chandrasana

FIGURE 10-22:
Ardha
Chandrasana,
with top hand
on hip

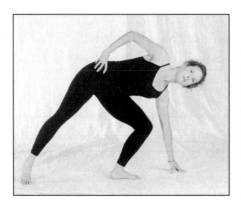

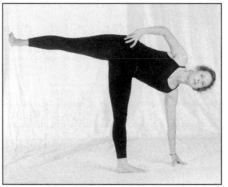

Keep lengthening both sides of the body from the hips to the armpits, paying particular attention to the left side. Stretch from the coccyx to the crown of the head. Look straight ahead, and see if you can turn your body to face forwards. Firm the bottom hip under the top hip so the hips become stacked. Breathe! Root the left foot into the floor and stay in the pose for several breaths.

FIGURE 10-23:
Ardha
Chandrasana,
with arm
raised

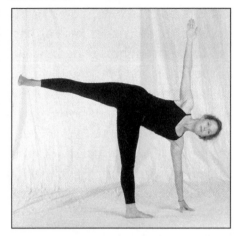

See if you can extend your right arm up, palm facing forward (SEE FIGURE 10-23). Otherwise, keep the hand on the hip. Smile! Remember that the pose is called half moon. The moon gracefully appears and (seemingly) disappears from the sky so gracefully and effortlessly. It seems to float in the sky. Can you achieve this graceful floating quality in Ardha Chandrasana, using your breath to link with the movement for a flowing sequence in and out of the pose?

FIGURE 10-24:
Ardha
Chandrasana,
with hand
on block

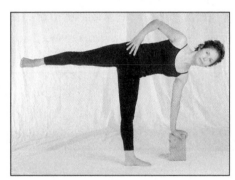

You can also practise this pose using a block under the bottom hand to help with balance and grounding (SEE FIGURE 10-24). Or practise with the back to the wall for support. This is a wonderful way to get accustomed to the mechanics and the flow and rhythm of the pose without worrying about balance.

In addition to the benefits of Trikonasana and Utthita Parsvakonasana, Ardha Chandrasana offers the following benefits:

· It helps balance asymmetry of the sides of the body.
· It strengthens muscles that are weak and stretches those that are tight.
· It elongates the spine.
· It strengthens the hips, legs, knees and foot arches.
· It stretches the hamstrings.

PARSVOTTANASANA

Parsvottanasana is an asymmetrical forward bend, which stretches each side of the body separately. The chest receives an intense stretch. Stand in Tadasana. Jump or walk the feet wide apart. Place the hands on the hips. Turn the left foot in 45° to 60°, and turn the right leg out. Inhale the breath, grounding the feet, lifting the arches and bringing the inhalation and extension all the way up the legs and the body. Lifting the ribs away from the hips, maintain the lift of the quadriceps and the hugging action of the leg muscles throughout the pose.

Exhale and turn to face your right leg. Place the hands in reverse prayer position, with palms together, fingers pointing up and the little fingers against behind the middle back. Revolve the left leg in its socket, turning the front thigh to face forward (without strain or force). Inhale and extend the spine, looking up (SEE FIGURE 10-25). Exhale and, bending from the hips, swing the body over the right leg (SEE FIGURE 10-26). Gaze at your toes. Lengthen from the crown of the head to the coccyx.

FIGURE 10-25:
Going into
Parsvottan-
asana

FIGURE 10-26:
Parsvottan-
asana

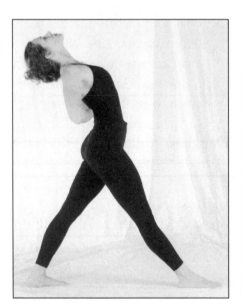
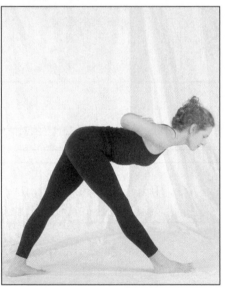

See if you can balance the forward action of the torso extending over the front leg by pulling your hips back and drawing the top of the thighs and the hamstrings behind you. Then you will be moving in two directions, creating space throughout the spine. If you only move forward, you will lose your balance and fall forward. If you can bend more deeply in the hips and maintain the length created in the spine, bring your head towards your shin (SEE FIGURE 10-27).

FIGURE 10-27: Parsvottan-asana, bent deeply

FIGURE 10-28: Parsvottan-asana, using a chair

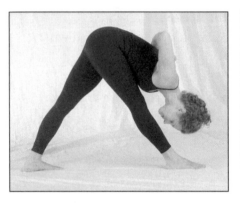 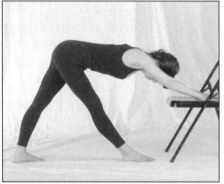

Try to keep the feet grounded and draw the thigh bones into the hip socket. Simultaneously level the hips by pulling the outer right hip back and releasing the left hip forward to help you turn the hips even more. Stay in the pose for a few breaths, and then come back up by pressing strongly into the feet with strong, muscle-hugging legs and a long spine. Repeat on the other side. Place the back heel on the wall if you need additional support.

FIGURE 10-29: Parsvottan-asana, using blocks

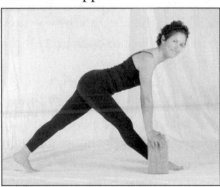

You can also practise Parsvottanasana by placing the hands (with stretched, straight arms) on a chair seat as you come into the pose (SEE FIGURE 10-28). Focus on elongating the spine and keeping it concave.

Or, as you come into the pose, place the hands on blocks on either side of the front foot (SEE FIGURE 10-29). Lengthen the arms down into the hands and up into the arm sockets, providing support for the upper body and stability in the pose.

The benefits of Parsvottanasana include the following:

- It improves balance and coordination.
- It lengthens the hamstrings and the back side of the body.
- It opens the hips.
- It tones the abdomen.
- It cools the brain and calms the nerves.
- It relieves arthritis of the neck, shoulders, elbows and wrists.
- It improves digestion.
- It tones the liver and spleen.
- It reduces menstrual pain when practised before and after (not during) menstruation.

PRASARITA PADOTTANASANA

Prasarita Padottanasana is a wide-legged forward bend that fully stretches the back and opens the hamstring muscles. Over time, the back muscles and the hamstrings will release more and more.

Stand in Tadasana and jump the feet wide apart. Place the hands on the hips. Make the feet parallel to each other (SEE FIGURE 10-30). Spread the toes as you press the soles of the feet down and lift the inner and outer arches up. Rebound the action up the legs, lifting the kneecaps, firming the quadriceps and hugging the leg muscles to the bone. Lengthen the sides of the body away from the hands (on the hips) all the way up to the armpits. Press the shoulder blades into the back to open and lift the chest. Breathe and expand the lungs out to the side ribs.

Inhale the breath. As you exhale, fold forward from the hips, maintaining the length of the spine you have just created. Place your fingertips on the floor (or your palms, if flexible) shoulder-width apart, either in line with the toes or in front of the toes (SEE FIGURE 10-31). The arms are fully stretched, with the upper arms drawn up into the shoulder sockets. Keep the length of the spine. The front, back, and sides of the body remain elongated, and the back is concave.

FIGURE 10-30:
Preparation for
Prasarita
Padottan-asana

FIGURE 10-31:
Prasarita
Padottan-asana

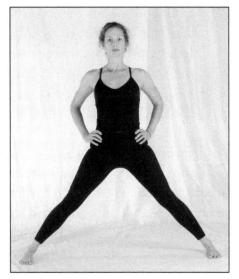

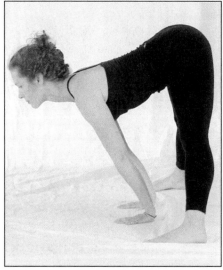

FIGURE 10-30:
Preparation for
Prasarita
Padottan-asana

FIGURE 10-31:
Prasarita
Padottan-asana

FIGURE 10-32:
Prasarita
Padottan-asana

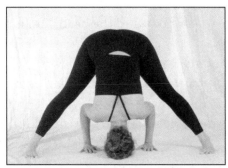

Look straight ahead, lengthening into the crown of the head and into the coccyx. Keep breathing, and on an exhalation, fold deeper into the hip crease and let the head and spine hang down as the coccyx lifts up. Let the elbows bend back toward the legs as the palms come down to the floor.

Maintain the feet and leg action throughout the posture and keep the weight in the legs, so the spine can be free. Observe whether you are locking (hyperextending) the knees (SEE FIGURE 10-32).

Stay for a few breaths, breathing fully without strain. Then inhale and look forward, straightening the arms and again lengthening into the crown of the head and the coccyx (SEE FIGURE 10-31). Exhale. Place the hands on the hips and stamp the feet down, activating the legs even more. Lift the shoulders up and the coccyx slightly away from the floor, and look forwards. Create a long spine to come out of the posture. Release the arms down to the sides.

FIGURE 10-33:
Prasarita
Padottan-
asana, using
blocks

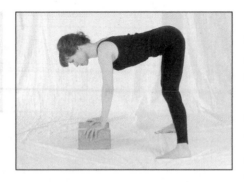

If your hands do not easily make it to the floor, due to tight hamstrings and a tight lower back, place the hands on two blocks (SEE FIGURE 10-33). Lengthen the spine and work the legs. If the hamstrings are very tight, soften the knees, allowing them to bend. Work on elongating the spine. Practise this way for a while. As the hamstrings begin to ease, press down through the feet and draw up the kneecaps and quadriceps to create a fully stretched leg. This action will help free the spine.

The benefits of Prasarita Padottanasana include the following:

- It opens the hips.
- It increases blood flow to the upper body and the head, and is good preparation for the headstand.
- It fully stretches the hamstring muscles.
- It strengthens the adductor (inner thigh) muscles.
- It improves digestion.
- It's a good substitute for those unable to do the headstand.

UTTANASANA

Uttanasana is a standing-forwards bend – an intense stretch of the hamstring muscles and a lengthening and strengthening of the back muscles and the spine. Stand in Tadasana. Inhale the breath, root down onto the feet, stretch up through the legs and elongate the spine as you contract the kneecaps and the quadricep muscles to help the hamstrings lengthen. Firm the thigh muscles as you lift up through the crown of the head.

Roll the upper inner thighs and groin back, keeping the lower back broad. Draw the shoulder blades into the back to lift and open the chest. Maintain active yoga feet, a strong lift of the inner groin and legs. Actively lift and stretch your side ribs and spine up and over as you exhale and bend forward, folding at the hips.

FIGURE 10-34:
Uttanasana

FIGURE 10-35:
Uttanasana,
using blocks

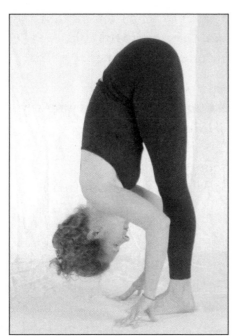
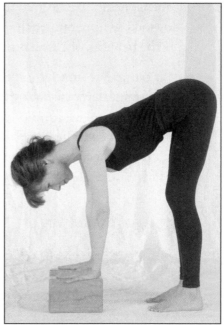

Let the arms come down towards the floor. Place the fingertips on the floor in front of the feet (SEE FIGURE 10-34). The legs draw up so the spine can release down. Breathe and allow the effects of gravity to release the back muscles, spine and head down. Contract the kneecaps and the quadricep muscles to help the hamstrings lengthen. Broaden the backs of the calves and the backs of the thighs.

When you are ready to come up, press the feet down and keep the legs really active, so that the strength of the thigh muscles supports the stretch of the hamstring. This will prevent the feeling of locking the knees (hyperextension of the knees, pressing the knees back). Look forwards, lengthening the crown of the head and the coccyx away from each other. Inhale and come up with a concave back.

You can practice Ardha Uttanasana (see page 130) until you feel ready to move on to Uttanasana. If the hamstrings are tight, use a block under each hand (SEE FIGURE 10-35). The knees can also be bent, allowing the spine to lengthen and the spinal muscles to strengthen.

You may want to widen the distance between the feet to hip width or a little wider. Turn the toes in and come into the pose. Turning the toes in deepens the hip crease, making it easier to bend from the hips and allowing the upper inner thighs and the groin to roll back.

The benefits of Uttanasana include the following:

·   It reduces stomach discomfort.
·   It strengthens the back muscles and the hamstrings intensely.
·   It relieves mental and physical exhaustion.
·   It slows down the heartbeat.
·   It tones the liver, spleen and kidneys.
·   It decreases abdominal and back pains during menstruation.

ARDHA UTTANASANA

Ardha Uttanasana is the standing half-forwards bend, using a chair. Place the hands on the top sides of a chair back and press the hands into the back. As the hands root into the chair back, stretch the arms back into the shoulder socket. Remember: for every action there is an equal and opposite reaction. The elbows are firm and straight. Continue lengthening from the shoulders to the buttock bones, making the sides of the waist long. Keep the shoulder blades in contact with the back body and back ribs. This stabilizes the shoulder joint and helps to open the chest. Even in a forward bend the chest remains open and the spine remains long. This action will help keep the spine happy, whereas the legs should do the most work in the pose so the spine receives the action.

The body is parallel to the floor, with the head between the arms. The neck and head are in line with the spine. The crown of the head stretches forward as the coccyx lengthens back. The heels are in line with the buttocks, and the feet are hip-width (or wider) apart. Tight hamstrings require a wider leg stance. Maintain active yoga feet and legs.

Make sure that you are not pressing the shoulders or front ribs down in an effort to open the body. You want a long line of stretch from the fingertips to the buttocks and from the buttocks to the heels. If the body hangs from a joint (for example, shoulder, hyperextended knees, floating ribs), then the line of energy will be broken and the extension will occur in the tendons and ligaments instead of the stomach or the muscles.

Broaden the lower back by spreading the buttock bones away from each other, letting the inner thighs hug the thigh bones. Pull the hips and tops of the thighs back towards the middle of the room to create even more length in the spine.

Feel the terrific space and length in the torso and the back of the legs. Stay for a few breaths and enjoy the space you have created in your body. This pose also can be done as a restorative pose for resting the back, by resting the front of the torso on a table or counter.

The benefits of Ardha Uttanasana include the following:

· It fully stretches the back side of the body.
· It lengthens the spine and teaches alignment.

During the first trimester of pregnancy, standing poses should be done against the wall and only for short periods of time to avoid dizziness and fatigue. Vigorous standing postures are not appropriate during pregnancy. Consult your doctor.

UTKATASANA

Utkatasana, the chair pose or fierce warrior, is a pose that teaches you how to bend well at the hip, knee and ankle joints. It is a good warm-up pose because it stretches the arms over the head and works major muscles of the legs. The hips move down and crease, as if to sit, while the torso and arms lengthen upwards, creating a dynamic stretch. It is a wonderful pose for developing stamina and endurance, and is great preparation for skiing. Remember to listen to your body and the breath, and come out of the pose when it is time to rest.

Stand in Tadasana and separate the feet hip width apart. Bend the hips as if to sit down. Also bend the knees and the ankles as deeply as (comfortably) possible. Ground the feet and slightly draw your weight back into your heels, so they receive most of the weight. This makes the action felt in the thighs rather than the lower back, since the legs are doing the work, and it is better for the health of the back.

Pressing down into the active yoga feet, bring the buttocks down, inhale and stretch the arms up. Lift the frontal hip bones up away from the thighs. The thighs will do most of the work in the pose – there will be sensation to confirm this. The area around the ankles will feel a good amount of stretch and action. The groin and abdomen remain soft and recede into the body.

Lengthen into the fingertips, connecting this action with the lifting and stretching of the side ribs, while drawing the upper arm bones back into the socket. Lift the top chest to help move the shoulder blades into the back. Look straight ahead and breathe. Feel the expansion of the chest area. Monitor your breath, looking for ease and smooth regularity of the inhalation and exhalation. To come out of the pose, exhale and release the arms down to the sides as you press the feet into the floor and lift the kneecaps and quadriceps to lengthen the legs back into Tadasana.

You can also perform this pose standing with your feet 46cm (18in) away from the wall with your back to the wall. Bring your feet thigh-distance or a little further away from the wall. Bend the knees, hips and ankles and come into Utkatasana with the back supported on the wall. Work your feet. Feel the thigh action and the softening of the groins and abdomen. Stretch the arms actively and observe the stretch and opening of the ribs and the side body. Lift the top chest. Stay as long as possible and then allow the back to come off the wall. The buttocks will touch the wall as you extend the arms in Utkatasana.

The classic pose is done with the feet together. Balance will be more of a focus throughout the posture. (Having feet apart ensures the openness and broadness of the lower back.)

The benefits of Utkatasana include the following:

· It strengthens the back, legs, ankles, shoulders, and arms.
· It eases shoulder stiffness and expands the chest.
· It lifts the diaphragm and gently massages the heart.

If you suffer from knee pain, try to balance the action of the feet, placing equal weight on both sides of the feet and strongly lifting the inner and outer arches. Turn the toes out slightly. If this does not help, come out of the pose.

CHAPTER 11
Seated Poses

Seated poses are calming and quietening, allowing you to reflect and be absorbed into the pose, infused with the breath and prana, and refreshed from the pose. In the *Yoga Sutra*, it is said that one should be relaxed, alert and focused, steady and comfortable in a pose. In seated postures the buttock bones and the legs are the foundation from which extension, vitality and suppleness of the spine are made possible.

DANDASANA

Dandasana, the staff pose, is the fundamental seated posture. It is to sitting poses what Tadasana is to standing postures. Dandasana teaches the foundation and basic principles crucial to correct seated postures.

Sit evenly on the buttock bones with the legs outstretched and together, in front of you. Place your hands slightly behind the hips and press the fingertips down into the floor as you lightly lift the buttocks off the floor. The buttocks will hover over the floor. As you press the fingertips down, stretch the arms up into their sockets. Firm the arm muscles to the bones without tensing the shoulders and neck. This action will stretch and lift the sides of the body and lengthen the spine.

Lightly lower the buttocks to the floor. Press down through the buttock bones and feel the rebounding action going up the torso, lifting and lengthening the spine out of the pelvis. Accentuate this by extending up through the sides of the body. Move the shoulder blades into the back.

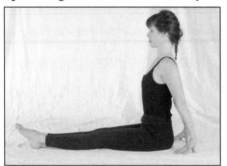

FIGURE 11-1:
Dandasana

Maintain the pressing down of the fingertips and stretching of the arms to support the torso and elongate the spine. Breathe! Broaden the collarbones and lift the sternum (breastbone), opening the top chest and keeping the shoulder blades into the back to support the opening of the chest.

Press the back of the legs and the buttock bones firmly into the floor for your foundation. Avoid pressing just the knees down to lengthen the legs, because this creates hyperextension of the knees. The legs must lengthen and extend for the legs to press down onto the floor. Encourage the legs to stretch in two directions. Lengthen the legs into the active yoga feet. Firm the thighs and lift the kneecaps as the thigh bones draw into the hip sockets.

Throughout the pose, keep the centre of the back of the heel on the floor with the toes straight up. Have the hands by the hips, fingers facing forwards, lightly touching the floor, while supporting the elongation of the spine. Stretch up through the crown of the head (SEE FIGURE 11-1).

Gaze straight ahead with a soft but focused gaze. Reflect and watch your breath. How do you feel? Stay for several breaths or minutes, depending upon the ease and effort felt in the posture.

It can be helpful to sit on a folded blanket or two, to bring the pelvis to an upright, level position to maintain the natural curves of the spine (SEE FIGURE 11-2). Then it is easier to hinge forward from the hips. You can also widen the distance between the legs, or use a belt or strap for the feet while lifting the spine, or place the hands on blocks (SEE FIGURE 113).

FIGURE 11-2:
Dandasana,
while sitting on
folded blankets

FIGURE 11-3:
On blocks

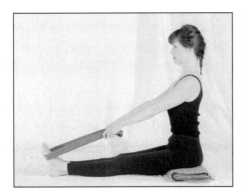
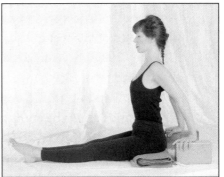

You can sit with the back against the wall for support. Bring the upper arm and the top of the shoulder blades back against the wall. This opens the chests, works the upper back muscles and draws the shoulder blades in to lift, open and support the chest. Sit facing the wall and press your active yoga feet into the wall, encouraging the legs to stretch fully in two directions (knee to heel and knee to hip). Continue pressing down through the buttock bones and fingertips while elongating the side body and spine.

The benefits of Dandasana include:

· It aligns the head, chest, pelvis and spine.
· It creates optimal space for the organs to function properly.
· It lengthens the spine.
· It strengthens back and chest muscles.
· It stretches the back of the legs.
· It tones the abdominal organs.
· It reduces heartburn and flatulence.

If you suffer from back pain, try ways to practise and gradually build up strength and endurance of your back muscles. Standing postures that fully stretch the legs must be practised for ease in the back as well as Supta Padangusthasana, which fully stretches the hamstrings while the back, which is supported by the floor, is not involved.

VAJRASANA

Vajrasana, the thunderbolt pose, is a great pose to do everyday. It is wonderful for the knees and stretches and opens the front of the ankle, shins, soles of the feet and backs of the legs. The feet benefit greatly in increased flexibility and development of the arches, which support and absorb and rebound the weight of the body.

Sit in Dandasana and come into a kneeling position with the spine upright and long. The shins and the front of the feet are on the floor. Plant the buttocks on the heels, place your palms on top of the thighs, exhale as you move the coccyx down and inhale as you lengthen up through the crown of the head. Elongate the spine and the sides of the body from the hips up to the armpits. Lift and open the top chest and move the shoulder blades into the back. Diffuse the eyes, soften the throat, open and spread the diaphragm, and soften the stomach as you gaze straight ahead. While gazing you are looking and yet not looking, perceiving it all but seeing nothing, for the gaze is turned inward. Stay for several breaths, expanding and opening the ribcage, and then release.

You can place a folded blanket under the shins and knees for cushioning (SEE FIGURE 11-4). Or roll up a sock or a hand towel and put it under the front of the ankles to ease the stretch there. If the knees are uncomfortable, place a folded blanket in the knee crease (SEE FIGURE 11-5). If the buttocks do not reach the heels, sit on a folded blanket between the heels and the buttocks (SEE FIGURE 11-6). Instead of sitting on the front of the feet, tuck the toes under. This increases toe flexibility and stretches the skin on the soles of the feet and the back of the legs. You can also stretch the arches of your feet (SEE FIGURE 11-7). If you suffer from knee pain, and none of the modifications of the pose help, come out of the pose.

FIGURE 11-4:
Vajrasana with
a blanket
under the
shins

FIGURE 11-5:
With a blanket
between the
thighs and
calves

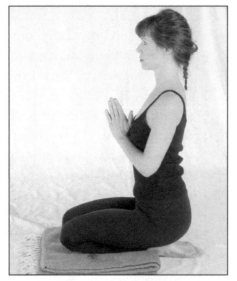
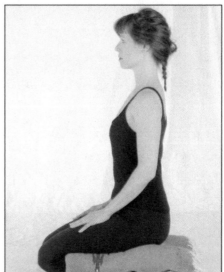

FIGURE 11-6:
Vajrasana, sit-
ting on a
blanket

FIGURE 11-7:
With toes
tucked under

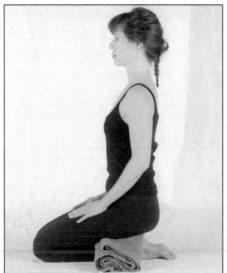
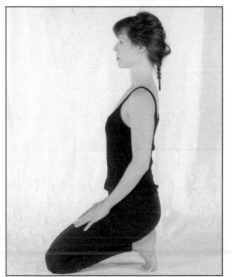

Vajrasana increases flexibility of ankles, knees and hips; strengthens
the arches; and helps digestion.

PARVATASANA

FIGURE 11-8:
Parvatasana,
using a belt

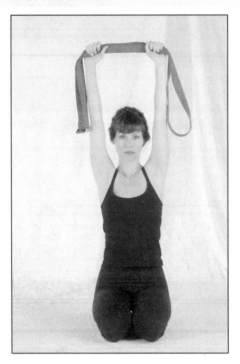

Parvatasana is the seated mountain pose. Sit in Vajrasana. Interlock your fingers and stretch your arms out in front of you. Draw the upper-arm bones back into their sockets, to stretch the arms fully. Turn the palms to face out and stretch into the palms. Inhale and bring the arms up over the head. Squeeze the upper arms in toward the head as the forearms stretch up. Elongate from the side ribs to the palms. Stay for several breaths and then release. Change the interlock of the fingers and repeat the pose. If your shoulders are stiff, use a belt to hold onto, instead of interlocking the fingers (SEE FIGURE 11-8). You can also practise any of the modifications for Vajrasana earlier in this chapter.

The benefits of Parvatasana include the following:

· It improves shoulder flexibility.
· It strengthens upper-back muscles.
· It opens the chest.
· It stretches the wrists and forearms.

If you suffer from shoulder pain, go easy and don't push the stretch. People with high blood pressure should not practise this pose, and those with cardiac disorders should not raise the arms over the head.

VIRASANA

Virasana is the hero's pose. Sit in Dandasana and come to a kneeling position. Separate the feet and sit down between them. The feet should touch each hip (as best you can). Ground the buttock bones, sitting evenly on them. Pressing down into the buttock bones, exhale, inhale and lengthen through the spine to the crown of the head. Feel the torso lengthen, creating space between the ribs and the hips. Place the palms on the thighs. Soften the stomach, groin and thighs as you breathe in the pose. Gaze softly ahead with your inward focused eyes, seeing but not seeing (SEE FIGURE 11-9).

FIGURE 11-9:
Virasana

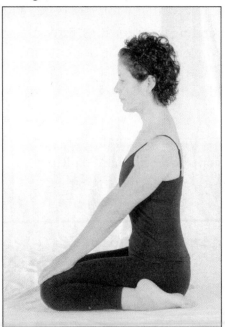

To come out of the pose, carefully bring one leg forward at a time. Keep the knee bent and draw it into the chest, bringing the heel in toward the buttocks. Slowly outstretch the leg on the floor, pressing the heel forward. Sit in Dandasana. If the knees hurt, come out of the pose. If knee pain persists while using the following modifications, this pose is not for you at this time. Try practising Vajrasana instead.

If the buttocks don't reach the floor, sit on a block or a phone book for support and grounding (SEE FIGURE 11-10, p 138). To ease knee discomfort, put a folded blanket in the knee crease (as in Vajrasana) and then come into Virasana. Or roll a sock or hand towel for each knee and place it in the crease. For ankle discomfort, roll a sock or a hand towel and place it under the front of the ankle.

FIGURE 11-10:
Virasana with a
block under
the buttocks

FIGURE 11-11:
Adho Mukha
Virasana

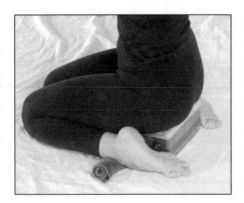
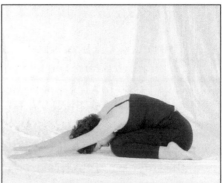

You can also try Adho Mukha Virasana as a forward bend. Widen the knees hip-width apart and, bending from the hips, extend the torso and arms forwards. Keep the buttock bones on the floor. Rest the forehead and hands on the floor (SEE FIGURE 11-11).

The benefits of Virasana include the following:

· It opens the knee joint.
· It stretches the shins and the fronts of the ankles.
· The arches are properly developed over time and daily practice.
· It's good for flat feet because it develops and strengthens the arches.
· It relieves calcaneal spurs through daily practice.
· It decreases pain of a broken, deviated or fused coccyx.
· It helps herniated discs.
· It improves circulation in the feet.
· It relieves gout.
· It decreases fullness in the stomach after meals.
· It helps create internal rotation of the thighs, important in backbends and forward bends.
· It decreases leg fatigue by increasing blood circulation in the legs.

You should never experience knee pain in a pose. If you do, try Vajrasana instead. Those with arthritis of the knees, cartilage tears and ligament problems should work with a qualified teacher. This pose is excellent for knees when done properly, under the supervision of a knowledgeable yoga instructor.

SUKHASANA

Sukhasana is the sitting pose we Westerners refer to as sitting cross-legged. According to Patanjali's *Yoga Sutras,* postures should be steady and comfortable. Sukhasana is such a posture, well suited to meditation and breathing practices.

Begin in Dandasana and cross the legs at the ankles. With your hands, roll the inner thighs down to the floor and then draw the flesh of the buttocks diagonally back behind you to broaden your base and lengthen the groin. Ground the buttock bones equally as you exhale. Inhale and let the thighs release down to the floor. Lengthen up through the sides of the body. Place the hands by the hips and, as in Dandasana, lift the buttocks off the floor slightly and then lightly place them back down, maintaining a long torso. Lift and expand the chest.

Put the palms on top of the thighs, closer to the hips. Lift and open the top chest. Gaze straight ahead for several breaths. Release the pose, change the cross of the legs and do Sukhasana again.

FIGURE 11-12:
Sukhasana on a
blanket

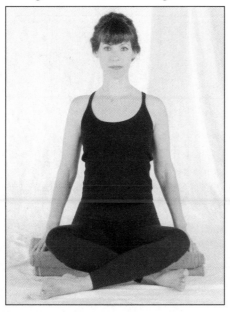

You can also practise this pose while sitting on one or several blankets so the knees and hips are level with each other and the pelvis is in a level, upright position, maintaining the natural curves of the spine (SEE FIGURE 11-12). This correctly feeds the thigh bones into the hip sockets for stabilization and support of the pelvis. (Don't fret if your knees and hips are not level. It is a goal to work toward on the journey of yoga.) If the knees are high above the floor, this won't work. Just sit higher.

You can also try sitting in Sukhasana with the back against a wall for support. Or see if you can cross the legs at the shins. Crossing at the shins, not the ankles, provides a more intense opening of the hips. Observe whether you can experience comfort and ease doing the pose this way. If not, return to crossing at the ankles.

Sukhasana bends and opens the knees and externally rotates and increases flexibility of the hips.

If you have knee pain, it may be better to sit in a chair, with the feet flat on the floor, directly under the knees, and the spine erect. Or try sitting in Vajrasana or Virasana instead.

GOMUKHASANA

Gomukhasana is the cow's head pose. Bend the right leg over the left leg, and swing the right leg to the left side with the right knee over the left knee. The right shin and foot are by the left side. The knees are at the mid-line of the body and the toes are pointing back (SEE FIGURE 11-13).

FIGURE 11-13:
Gomukhasana
legs

FIGURE 11-14:
Gomukhasana
arms and legs

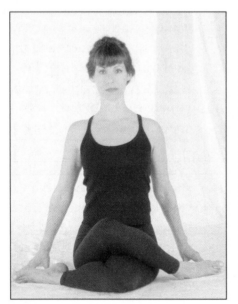
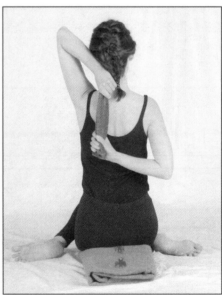

Press down evenly into the buttock bones and rebound the stretch up through the torso, stretching the stomach, lower back and ribs away from the grounding action of the buttocks. Extend the left arm up. Wrap the right arm behind the body. Bend the elbows and see if you can clasp the fingers of each hand together on the back, between the shoulders. If not, use a strap (SEE FIGURE 11-14). Stretch the elbows away from each other and pull the fingers as if trying to draw them apart.

FIGURE 11-15: Gomukhasana legs from all fours FIGURE 11-16: Gomukhasana legs from all fours

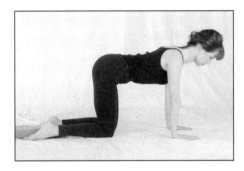 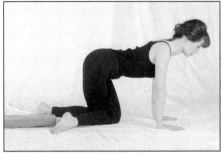

Bring the left arm up and back, with the inner arm next to the left ear. Draw the right shoulder back to bring the shoulder blade into the body. Expand the ribcage with the breath, and lengthen the sides of the body equally. Lift and broaden the collarbones.

FIGURE 11-17: Gomukhasana legs

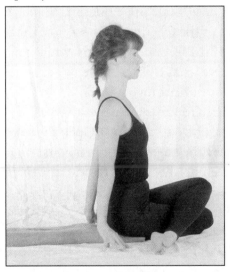

Remain in the pose for several breaths and then release the arms and legs back into Dandasana. Do the pose on the other side, changing the cross of the legs and the position of the arms.

Do not force the leg position. If it is uncomfortable, try the modifications in this section. If the modifications don't help, sit in Virasana or Vajrasana, and do the Gomukhasana arms.

As a modification, you can sit on one or several blankets or a block to bring the pelvis to a level, upright position. Another way to come into Gomukhasana legs is to start on your hands and knees (SEE FIGURE 11-15), cross the legs at the knees (SEE FIGURE 11-16, p 141), and sit back between the shins (SEE FIGURE 11-17, p 141).

The benefits of Gomukhasana include the following:

- It stretches and broadens the lower back.
- It opens hip joints and stretches hip muscles.
- It increases leg flexibility.
- It increases shoulder flexibility and relieves shoulder stiffness.
- It strengthens the muscles of the upper back.

Remember to distinguish between 'good' pain and 'bad' pain. Good pain is from opening a tight area, while bad pain may be injurious to ligaments, tendons and muscle, and is to be avoided. If you suffer from knee pain, arthritic knees, torn cartilage or ligament damage, try the modifications to the pose. If the modifications don't help, sit in Virasana or Vajrasana. If you have hip pain, stop and sit in Sukhasana or Vajrasana.

BADDHA KONASANA

Baddha Konasana is the cobbler pose. Start in Dandasana. Bend the knees out to the side and join the soles of the feet. Press the soles of the feet together, pressurizing the balls of the feet and the heels, while you peel the toes away from each other. Observe what this feels like. What actions do you observe in the legs? Check your breathing.

Using the hands, draw the feet in towards the pelvis to where it is comfortable. Let the thighs release down to the floor. Open the soles of the feet with your hands, as if they were the pages of an open book. Place the fingertips on the floor behind the hips. Press into the fingertips and stretch up through the arms. This will lift and lengthen the spine and the sides of the body. Inhale and press into the buttock bones (SEE FIGURE 11-18). Elongate the spine all the way to the crown of the head. Exhale fully and lift the top chest, keeping the shoulder blades on the back. Remain in this position for several breaths. Join the knees together and come into Dandasana. You may want to sit with the back against the wall to give yourself some support.

FIGURE 11-18:
Baddha
Konasana

FIGURE 11-19:
Baddha
Konasana with
blocks

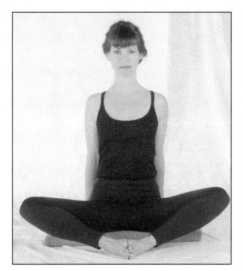
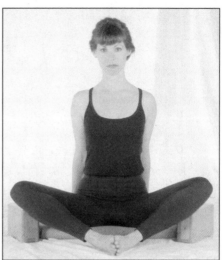

You can also try this pose sitting on a blanket to maintain an upright, level pelvis. Place the rounded corner of the folded blanket to face forward. Sit down with the rounded corner under the pubis. This will allow the thighs and groin to release further down to the floor. Or place a rolled-up blanket or a block under each knee for support and relaxation of the thigh muscles (SEE FIGURE 11-19).

Bring the feet further forward into the star pose. This will enable the knees and thighs to release further to the floor. Fold forwards from the hips, maintaining a long spine and keeping the buttock bones planted on the floor (SEE FIGURE 11-20).

FIGURE 11-20:
Star pose

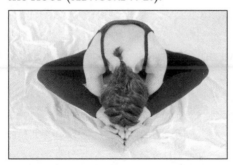

You can also try placing the hands behind you, with the fingertips on the floor, as you come forward (SEE FIGURE 11-21, p 146). This is a great way to learn how to bend forward from the hips without rounding the shoulders and upper back.

FIGURE 11-21:
Baddha
Konasana with
fingertips
behind hips

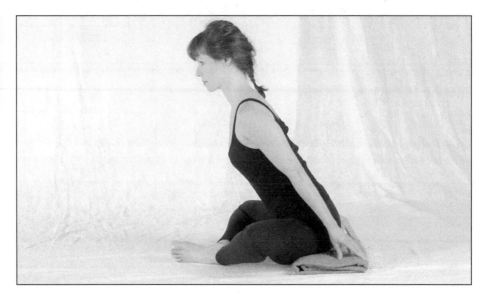

The benefits of Baddha Konasana include the following:

· It stretches the inner thighs and groins.
· It opens the pelvis and lower back.
· It reduces sciatic pain.
· It maintains the health of the kidneys, prostate, ovaries and bladder.
· It is a wonderful pose for pregnancy, helping with delivery and diminishing varicose veins.
· It eases menstrual discomfort.
· It is recommended for pranayama and meditation practices.

If you suffer from knee pain and none of the modifications help, refrain from doing the pose and try Upavistha Konasana.

NAVASANA

Navasana is the boat pose. Start in Dandasana. Bend the knees and lift the feet off the floor, raising the legs to 60° as you balance on the front of the buttock bones. Simultaneously extend the arms forwards. Lengthen into the fingertips and draw the upper arm bones back into their sockets

(SEE FIGURE 11-22). This will stabilize and support the lifting and opening of the upper body. Make the feet and knees active, extend through the heels to stretch the backs of the leg, and let the thigh bones draw into the hip sockets to support and stabilize the pelvis. Keep the elbows as firm as the knees. Elongate the spine and lift the top chest, looking forward. The abdomen is soft, not tense. The lower back (sacrum) is lifting as it comes into the body. Try not to round the back or lean back. Stay for several smooth breaths and release.

FIGURE 11-22:
Navasana

FIGURE 11-23:
Navasana with
knees bent,
feet
on floor

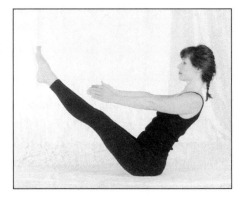 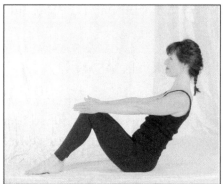

You can also try keeping the feet on the floor with knees bent (SEE FIGURE 11-23). Or keep the knees bent and hands holding onto knees, with the feet raised (SEE FIGURE 11-24). Or try Navasana with a belt around your feet. Hold onto the straps of the belt with each hand, maintaining a long spine and outstretched legs (SEE FIGURE 11-25).

FIGURE 11-24:
Navasana with
knees bent,
hands clasping
knees

FIGURE 11-25:
With belt
around feet

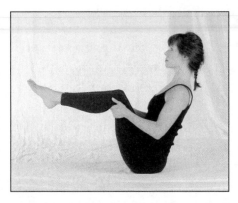 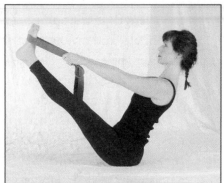

If you have a weak lower back, go easy on it and try some of the modifications listed here.

The benefits of Navasana include the following:

- It tones the kidneys.
- It trims the waistline and the abdomen.
- It tones the abdominal muscles.
- It strengthens the spinal muscles.
- It stimulates the intestines.
- It stimulates the thyroid gland, increasing the body's metabolic rate.

JANU SIRSASANA

Janu Sirsasana is the head-to-knee pose. Begin by sitting in Dandasana. Bend the right leg out to the side. Holding onto the back of the knee, draw the knee back to a comfortable position. Place the sole of the foot by the inner left thigh. The left leg is extended as in Dandasana, with the centre of the back heel on the floor. The left foot is actively spreading, the inner and outer arches are lifting, and the balls, joints of the toes, and heel are stretching forward.

Turn the body to face the left leg. Clasp the outer foot or hold onto the outer shin with the hands. Turn the navel to face the inner left leg. Press down evenly with the buttock bones, the back of the left leg, and the right thigh. Lengthen up through the sides of the body. Draw the upper-arm bones back into the sockets to open and lift the top chest. Enhance this action as you make the back concave, which creates more length in the spine.

Inhale, and on the exhalation bend from the hips and extend the body out over the extended left leg. Lift the ribs away from the hips. If you are more flexible, the arms may bend with the elbows out to the sides, causing the chest to remain wide.

If the extension of the spine is going well and there is ease in the pose, clasp the hands around the left foot, extend the arms and elongate the torso further as you exhale (SEE FIGURE 11-26). Rest the head on the left leg or a bolster or folded blanket.

Rounding the back and collapsing the front body indicates that you have gone into the flexibility of the spine and have skipped the stretch of the hamstrings. The spine is no longer elongated. Start again. Sit up and reaffirm the long spine. This is where you belong in the pose for now. Remain in the pose for several breaths. Come up and bring the right knee back to the centre and then the right leg into Dandasana. Repeat on the other side.

FIGURE 11-26:
Janu Sirsasana

FIGURE 11-27:
With belt and long spine

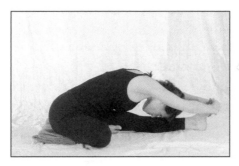 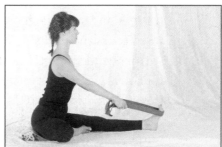

You can also try wrapping a belt around the ball of the outstretched foot (SEE FIGURE 11-27). Hold onto the belt without creating tension (no white knuckles!). Press the balls of the feet against the belt and lengthen the heel forward.

FIGURE 11-28:
Janu Sirsasana with belt and block under knee

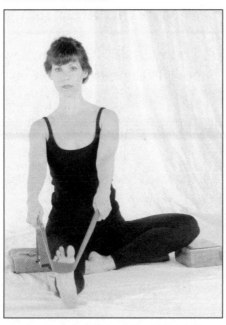

Or try placing a block or a folded blanket under the bent knee for support, if the knee is off the floor (SEE FIGURE 11-28). This will relax the groin and thigh muscles. For knee comfort, bring the bent knee foot further down the inner left leg, nearer to the left knee. The forehead can rest on folded blankets on the extended leg.

If you have knee pain, try the modifications to the pose. A block can be placed between the straight leg and the foot of the bent leg. If knee discomfort persists, don't attempt the pose.

Sometimes pain is felt in the sacroiliac joint when you're in this pose. The joint and its ligaments get overstretched due to faulty alignment. Great care must be taken not to overdo the pose, to set up properly for the pose and come out of the pose consciously (remember the continuum of a pose).

The benefits of Janu Sirsasana include the following:

- It tones the liver and spleen, improving digestion.
- It tones and stimulates the kidneys.
- It stretches the backside of the body and legs (one at a time), relieving stiffness and strengthening the leg muscles.
- It decreases stiffness in the shoulder, elbow, wrist and finger joints.
- It results in hip opening for the bent leg hip.
- It lengthens the spine.
- It increases knee flexibility.

TRIANG MUKHAIKAPADA PASCHIMOTTANASANA

Triang Mukhaikapada Paschimottanasana is the half-Virasana forward bend. Sit in Dandasana. Bend the left leg back, with the shin and the front of the foot on the floor. The left foot is next to the left hip, and the right leg stays in Dandasana.

Place the fingertips of each hand by your sides. Press them down as you inhale and root the buttock bones, and elongate the spine up through the crown of the head.

FIGURE 11-29:
Forehead
resting on
knee

FIGURE 11-30:
With belt
and blanket

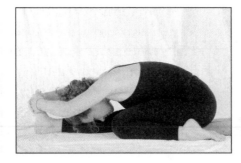 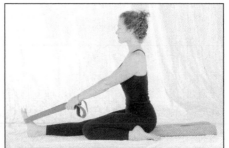

Clasp your hands around your foot. Lift the ribs off the hips. Continue grounding the buttock bones, the back of the right leg. and the left shin. Your forehead may rest on the right leg or above it (SEE FIGURE 11-29). Stay for several breaths and then come up and back into Dandasana. Repeat on the other side.

You can also try holding onto a belt strapped around the ball of the foot, and sitting on a blanket to elevate the pelvis and maintain a long spine (SEE FIGURE 11-30). The forehead can rest on a folded blanket on the outstretched leg (SEE FIGURE 11-31).

FIGURE 11-31:
**With head
support**

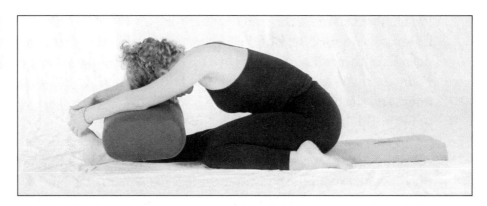

If you have knee pain, try one of the modifications. If knee pain continues, come out of the pose.

The benefits of Triang Mukhaikapada Paschimottanasana include the following:

· It opens the hips.
· It improves digestion.
· It creates flexibility in the knees.
· It develops foot arch on the bent-leg foot.
· It decreases swelling and discomfort from a sprained ankle.

Having trouble falling asleep? Try this technique developed by the Himalayan Institute. Watch your breath, through the nostrils. Gently slow down your exhalation until it's twice as long as the inhalation. Continue the two-to-one breathing ratio. Take 8 breaths lying on your back, 16 breaths lying on your right side, and 32 breaths lying on your left side.

PASCHIMOTTANASANA

Paschimottanasana is the seated straight-leg-forward bend. Sit in Dandasana on the centre of the back of your heels. Press the fingertips down on either side as you lengthen up through the sides of the torso. Maintain this as you clasp the feet with both hands. Ground the buttock bones and the back of the legs. Stretch your active yoga feet out as you draw the thigh bones back into the hip sockets.

Inhale, look up and lift up through the crown of the head, creating a concave spine. Keep the sternum lifted. Exhale as you bend forward from the hips and extend the body over the legs (SEE FIGURE 11-32). Lift the ribs away from the hips. Stay in the pose for several breaths. See if you can create more internal space as you inhale, and move deeper into the pose (if appropriate) with each exhale. Inhale up the front of the spine and exhale down the back. The forehead can rest on the legs or remain extended in the air. Gaze at the legs or the toes.

You can also try sitting on a folded blanket to keep the pelvis upright and neutral (SEE FIGURE 11-33). Place the fingertips behind the hips as you bend forward.

FIGURE 11-32:
Paschimottan-
asana

FIGURE 11-33:
With fingertips
behind hips for
spinal exten-
sion

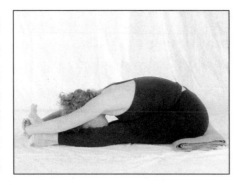
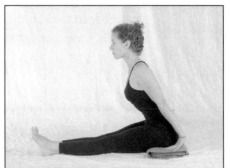

Or try using a strap around the balls of the feet. Hold onto the strap with each hand at a distance that allows ease in maintaining the length of the spine. Depending upon the flexibility of your hamstrings, either keep the knees bent slightly (SEE FIGURE 11-34) and focus on creating a long, concave spine, or stretch the legs fully (SEE FIGURE 11-35).

FIGURE 11-34:
Paschimottan-
asana
with belt
and knees
slightly bent

FIGURE 11-35:
With belt and
knees straight

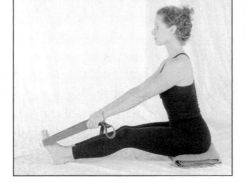
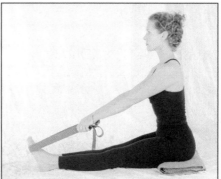

If you have very tight hamstrings, separate the legs and work with the modifications to this pose. Be patient. Over time and with practice, the hamstrings *will* release.

The benefits of Paschimottanasana include the following:

· It is an intense stretch for the back side of the body.
· It tones the abdominal organs.
· It improves digestion.
· It rejuvenates the spine.
· It calms and quietens the mind and the nervous system.
· It soothes the adrenal glands.
· It stimulates the ovaries, uterus and whole reproductive system.
· Once you are able to stay in the pose for several minutes, it gives the heart a good massage and replenishes the reproductive organs.

tips

If the spine presses out away from the back when forward bending, the front of the body will be shortened. When this happens, the lower back rounds and the stretch is felt in the back instead of the hamstrings, indicating that the pelvis is tilted backward. Sit on one or more blankets to elevate the buttocks and bring the pelvis to an upright, neutral position.

UPAVISTHA KONASANA

FIGURE 11-36:
Upavistha
Konasana,
intermediate

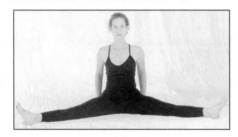

Upavistha Konasana is the seated wide-angle pose. Begin in Dandasana. Separate the legs at a comfortable, wide distance apart. Press the fingertips down by the sides of the body to lift and elongate the torso. Lift the ribcage off the hips. Root the centre of the back of the heels and the legs into the floor. The toes face the ceiling. Actively lengthen the legs in two directions, towards the feet and into the hips (SEE FIGURE 11-36). Breathe and be in the pose.

FIGURE 11-37:
Upavistha
Konasana

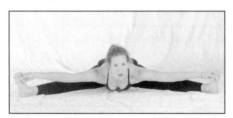

To go further in the posture, bend forwards from the hips and extend the body out and forward. Maintain the elongation of the front, sides and back of the body. Clasp the big toes or calves with your hands (SEE FIGURE 11-37). The buttock bones must remained grounded on the floor. The head may reach the floor or remain a little way off it.

You can also try sitting on a folded blanket. Place the rounded corner of the folded blanket to face forward. Sit down with the rounded corner under the pubis (SEE FIGURE 11-38). This will allow the thighs and groin to release further down to the floor. Wrap a belt around each foot and clasp one with each hand.

FIGURE 11-38:
Upavistha
Konasana with
belts

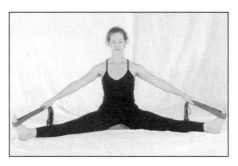

Benefits of Upavistha Konasana include: fully stretching the back of the body and the legs, toning the abdominal organs and improving the health of the reproductive organs by increasing circulation. It also balances the menstrual cycle, stimulates the ovaries and eases menstrual discomfort, while preparing the body for labour and delivery. In men, it tones and stimulates the prostate gland.

PARSVA UPAVISTHA KONASANA

Parsva Upavistha Konasana is the sideways wide-angle pose. Sit in Upavistha Konasana (refer to FIGURE 11-36). Turn the body to face the right leg. Place the right fingertips behind you and the left fingertips on the floor in front of the pubis. Press the fingertips down and ground the legs and the buttock bones as you inhale and lift the spine and sides of the body up. Exhale and gently revolve the body toward the right leg (SEE FIGURE 11-39). Continue inhaling and lengthening, and exhaling and revolving, for several breaths. Then carefully unwind back to the centre. Repeat on the other side.

FIGURE 11-39:
Parsva
Upavistha
Konasana

FIGURE 11-40:
With belt

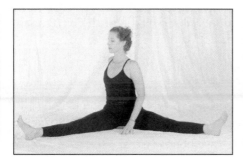

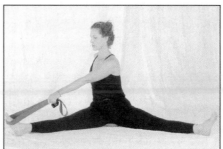

You can also try sitting on a folded blanket with the rounded corner under the pubis. Wrap a belt around the right foot and clasp it with the left hand (SEE FIGURE 11-40). The right fingertips are on the floor behind the right hips (SEE FIGURE 11-41). Pregnant women should limit the twisting action to the upper body and shoulders.

FIGURE 11-41:
Parsva
Upavistha
Konasana with
belt (back
view)

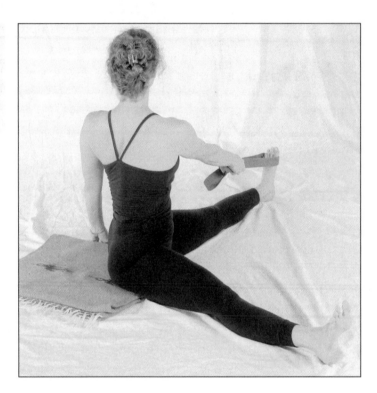

Parsva Upavistha Konasana relieves backaches, tones the abdominal organs, tones the kidneys, stimulates blood and lymph circulation and opens the hips.

Seated forward bends with a concave spine enhance the length of the spine. Pregnant women benefit from practising this way. People with lower back pain or weakness must be careful not to make the back concave, but instead focus on lengthening the spine. In time the back muscles are toned and strengthened, and the poses can be held longer.

CHAPTER 12
Twists

Twists are wonderful for releasing tension around the spine and for relieving backache and shoulder stiffness. Twists create a diagonal stretch and a revolving action, which initially elongates and wrings out waste in the muscles and organs and then infuses them with blood and nutrients. Twisting is vital to the health of the inter-vertebral discs, as they don't have a direct blood supply of their own.

BHARADVAJASANA ON CHAIR

Bharadvajasana is a sage twist. Sit sideways on a chair. The left side of the body is next to the back of the chair. Plant your feet flat on the floor with heels under knees. If the feet do not make it to the floor, bring the floor to you by placing a book or two under the feet.

FIGURE 12-1:
Bharadvaj-
asana on Chair

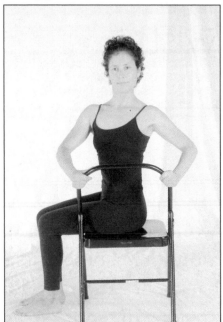

Hold onto the top sides of the chair back and bend the elbows wide apart to stretch and open the ribcage, making more room for the breath to enter. Press the buttock bones down into the chair seat as you inhale, and lengthen the sides of the body up. Exhale and gradually revolve the body around the spine, toward the back of the chair (SEE FIGURE 12-1). With every inhalation, create lift, extension and space in the body. After three or four breaths, unwind and return to the centre. Repeat on the other side.

If you're pregnant, concentrate the twisting action in the upper body and shoulders. During menstruation, the abdomen should remain soft and rested. Twists are not appropriate at this time.

The benefits of Bharadvajasana on Chair include the following:

·   It relieves arthritis of the lower back.
·   It improves digestion.
·   It alleviates rheumatism of the knees.
·   It tones the liver and kidneys.
·   It increases circulation to the abdominal organs.
·   It exercises the abdominal muscles.
·   It increases suppleness of spinal muscles.

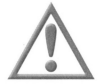

Twists must never be done aggressively, but gradually, lengthening and lifting the spine upon inhalation, and twisting and revolving on exhalation for several breaths, until no more movement is possible, otherwise the likelihood of injury is greatly increased. If you are leaning back and pressing down while twisting, this action could cause compression of the spine.

MARICYASANA III

Maricyasana III is another sage twist. Start in Dandasana. Press the fingertips of both hands onto the floor and lengthen the arms and torso. Bend the right knee and clasp both hands under the knee. Bring the knee into the chest and the heel to the right buttock bone. Firmly plant the right foot on the floor. Keep pressing the foot down throughout the posture. Extend through the left leg actively and press the back of the leg down.

Turn to the right. Wrapping the left arm around the right knee and hugging the leg into the body, place the right hand behind you. Re-create the length of the right arm and the extension of the right side of the body by pressing the fingertips down and drawing the arm up to the shoulder socket.

Inhale and extend the left arm up and, exhaling, bring the outside of the arm against the outside of the bent knees. Press the leg against the arm and the arm against the leg to help with the revolving action of the twist. Inhale the breath and extend the spine. Exhale and spiral the torso toward the right leg. Move the right knee forwards and bring the back ribs into the front ribs. Bend the left elbow and stretch the fingertips up to deepen the action and bring the shoulder blades onto the back (SEE FIGURE 12-2, p 158). Do this for several breaths, gently increasing the revolving of the spine and torso. Slowly release back to the centre, and repeat on the other side.

Instead of bringing the left arm to the outside of the right knee, you may want to try hugging the left arm around the right knee. Inhale, lengthen the spine and exhale, twisting while drawing the right leg into the body. You can also sit on a folded blanket to neutralize the pelvis. Place the back hand on a block (SEE FIGURE 12-3). This enhances the extension of the body on that side. You can also bend the elbows to increase the twisting action and open the chest.

FIGURE 12-2:
Maricyasana III

FIGURE 12-3:
Modified, with
arm
hugging bent
leg and back
hand on block

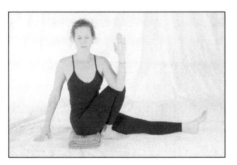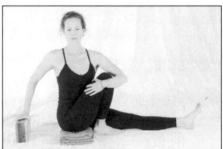

During pregnancy, the twist should be restricted to the upper body and shoulders. When menstruating, rest the abdominal area and keep it quiet.

The benefits of Maricyasana III include:

· It loosens the shoulders, lower back and hip.
· It increases energy levels.
· It improves the functioning of liver, spleen, pancreas, kidneys and intestines.
· It eases backache.
· It nourishes discs.

When twisting, do not let the head lead the way. There is a tendency to want to see where you're going, so the head and the eyes get overzealous. Twists spiral the spine and the body from the bottom up, like a corkscrew. The head is the last to turn and it learns from the chest.

JATHARA PARIVARTANASANA

Jathara Parivartanasana is the stomach-turning pose (SEE FIGURE 12-4). Lie down and bend the knees with the feet flat on the floor. Lift the feet away from the floor and bring the knees to the chest. Extend the arms horizontally out to the sides on the floor. Stack the knees and ankles and let the knees come down to the left, towards the floor at a right angle. The legs will hover over the floor, with the lower leg holding up the upper leg. Gaze up at the ceiling. Feel the stomach and ribs spiral toward the right. Maintain the length of the spine upon inhalation, twist on the exhalation and roll the right shoulder down toward the floor (without forcing). Stay in the pose for several breaths, deepening the twist. Then, bring the knees back to the centre and go to the other side.

FIGURE 12-4:
Jathara
Parivartan-
asana

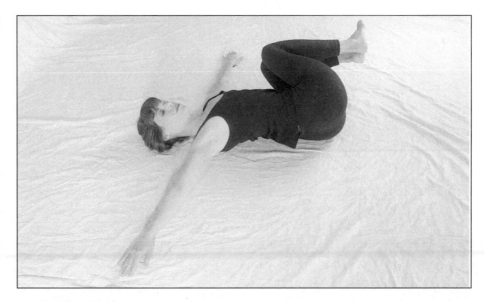

If hip mobility is restricted or the lower back is weak, place a folded blanket under the bottom leg for support.

Jathara Parivartanasana is not recommended during menstruation, as there is too much activity in the abdominal area. It is also unsuitable for pregnant women. This pose works too strongly on the abdomen, and it is also a flat, horizontal position, which may put too much pressure on major arteries.

The benefits of Jathara Parivartanasana include the following:

· It is a powerful, stimulating and wringing action for the waist, abdomen and lower back.
· It strengthens transverse and oblique abdominal muscles.
· It strengthens inner and outer thigh muscles.

CHAPTER 13
Supine and Prone Poses

S upine and prone poses stretch the abdomen and increase mobility of the spine. They strengthen the back, arms and legs, and open the hips and groin. Some of the poses are passive and restorative, while other postures are active and stimulating.

LEGS-UP-THE-WALL POSE

Legs-up-the-wall pose is a restorative, supine, inverted posture. Lie on your side with your buttocks close to the wall and your knees bent. Roll onto your back and swing the legs up the wall. Rest the backs of your legs on the wall and your back on the floor. Have your arms outstretched horizontally with the palms facing up. The eyes may close and soften. Breathe naturally and enjoy the relaxation and revitalization of the pose. To come out of the pose, bend the knees and with your feet, press yourself straight into the middle of the room. Roll onto your side, and, using your hands, press yourself up to a seated position.

Your knees can be slightly bent if it is too intense of a stretch for the hamstring muscles. The legs can also be separated wide apart.

Inversions are not recommended during menstruation. They are also not advised for people with a detached retina.

The benefits of the legs-up-the-wall pose include the following:

- It drains fluid from the legs.
- It softens the stomach and groin.
- It reverses the effects of gravity.
- It reverses the flow of blood and lymph.
- It rests the heart and the brain.
- It relieves tired legs.
- It revitalizes and relaxes.

When your legs are tired and aching, practise the legs-up-the-wall pose. This wonderful, mild inversion rests and revitalizes the legs. Circulation in the feet and legs is improved, and the legs feel great. Time spent in the pose is quiet time for your entire body and mind. Stay in the pose anywhere from 5 to 20 minutes and emerge refreshed!

SUPTA BADDHA KONASANA

Supta Baddha Konasana is the supported cobbler pose. Stack one to three vertically folded blankets one on top of the other behind you, with the narrower end a few centimetres away from your buttocks. Sit in Dandasana. Bend the knees out to the sides and join the soles of the feet together. Draw the heels in towards the pelvis at a comfortable distance for the knees and hips.

Place your hands on either side of the blankets and lower your back (keeping it extended) and head onto the blankets. Let your arms come out to the sides, with the palms facing up. They will be off the blankets.

Close your eyes. Relax completely. This is a wonderful restorative posture. Stay in the pose for 5 to 10 minutes, depending upon your comfort level. Observe your breath and the expansion of the torso upon inhalation and the contraction of the body on exhalation.

To come out of the pose, bring your knees together and carefully roll off the blankets onto your right side. Press your hands down to bring yourself to a seated position.

It may be necessary to place a folded blanket under your head, so your chin is neither pressing into your chest nor sticking up in the air. Your chin can be level with your forehead or a little lower. You want to retain the natural (concave) curve of the neck. Your legs can be propped up with additional blankets or blocks for extra support (SEE FIGURE 13-1).

For pregnant women, lying flat is not recommended. Instead, stack the blankets like stairs, to allow the torso to lie on an incline.

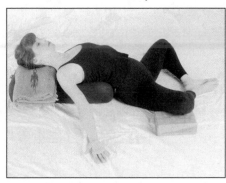

FIGURE 13-1:
Supta Baddha
Konasana

If you have lower back pain, come out of the pose and readjust the height of the blankets. See if this helps. Placing support under the thighs may ease the back. If you have knee pain, place support under the knees. Adjust the distance of the heels from the groin, creating a wider angle with the knees.

Or put a block between the feet, which takes the action out of the knees and places it into the hips. If pain persists, do not stay in the pose.

The benefits of Supta Baddha Konasana include the following:

- It eases menstrual discomfort.
- It opens the chest, abdomen, pelvis, inner thighs and groin.
- It deepens the breath.
- It's beneficial for the health of the ovaries and the prostate gland.
- It regulates blood pressure.
- It relieves varicose veins and sciatica.
- It helps a prolapsed uterus.
- It tones the kidneys.

SUPTA VIRASANA

Sit in Virasana with the feet on either side of the hips and the soles of the feet facing up. Stretch and spread your toes and the soles of your feet. Roll your inner thighs slightly down to the floor while spreading your buttock bones away from the coccyx, or turn the calves out. Have two to four vertically folded blankets, one on top of the other, placed behind your buttocks. Place the palms down on either side of the blankets, and lengthen the spine out of the pelvis. Rest on the elbows, as the body lowers onto the blankets (SEE FIGURE 13-2).

FIGURE 13-2:
Supta Virasana

FIGURE 13-3:
Preparation for
Supta Virasana

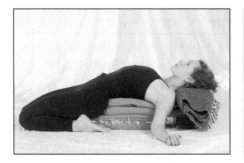
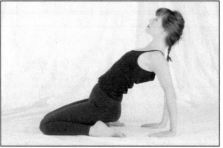

Remain in the pose up to five minutes, depending upon your level of comfort and ease. This is another great restorative pose. To come out of the pose, press the elbows and forearms down on either side of the blankets, and come up with the chest lifted. Carefully extend one leg at a time.

You can also practise this pose with your arms overhead with hands holding onto the opposite elbows, or extend your arms horizontally out to the sides.

Also try sitting in Virasana and placing the hands on the floor (fingers facing forwards) behind you, on the floor (SEE FIGURE 13-3). Press the hands down for foundation and grounding while you lift the chest. Feel the shoulder blades come into the back and the upper back muscles firm in to support the lift and opening of the chest.

Alternatively, place padding under the shins. Put a folded blanket in the knee crease to open and ease the knees, as in Virasana (FIGURE 11-10, p 138). Sit on some support if the buttocks don't reach the floor, as in Virasana. Place a rolled up sock or hand towel under the front of the ankles as in Virasana. Use as many folded blankets as necessary to be comfortable. Blankets can be stacked like stairs for gradual, elevated support. This is an excellent way for pregnant women to do the pose. Put a folded blanket under the head and neck to ensure proper alignment of the neck (chin neither tilting up or down into chest).

If you have knee pain, be very cautious. This may not be a good pose for you at this time. Try the modifications in this section. If knee pain continues, come out of the pose. If you have problems with cartilage or osteoarthritis of the knees, or suffer from cardiac disorders, this pose is not recommended. If you have lower back pain, be very cautious. Try the modifications, and if pain persists, do not stay in the pose.

The benefits of Supta Virasana include the following:

- It stretches the abdomen, waist, back, and front of thighs.
- It improves digestion.
- It opens the lungs and allows for easier breathing, providing some relief from asthma.
- It relieves menstrual discomfort.
- It reduces inflammation of the knees.
- It relieves pain in the legs and rests them.
- It enhances resistance to infection.
- It develops arches and helps correct flat feet.

The next time you've had too much to eat, help yourself feel better by practising Supta Virasana. Supta Virasana allows the front of the body, which houses the digestive organs, to receive a good stretch, making proper room and space for food assimilation and elimination. Energy channels located in this area are stimulated, creating balanced energy flow and improving digestion.

URDHVA PRASARITA PADASANA

Urdhva Prasarita Padasana is the upwards spread-out foot pose. Lie down with your arms by your sides. Exhale and bring the arms over your head, elbows firm and fingers stretched. Feel the stretch all the way from the hips to the fingertips and from the hips to the feet. Activate the feet and knees, and firm the legs.

Exhale and raise the legs to 90° (SEE FIGURE 13-4). Lengthen the lower back to the legs, and draw the thigh muscles up toward the hips. Lengthen the back of the legs to the heels, by stretching the heels away from the body. Press into the feet. Ground the outer hips down. Keep the eyes, throat and abdomen soft throughout the posture. Hold the pose for several seconds.

FIGURE 13-4:
Legs at 90°

FIGURE 13-5:
Legs at 60°

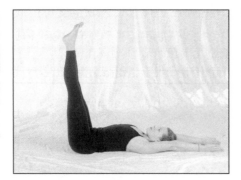
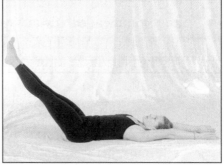

Then exhale and lower the legs to 60°, following the above actions for a few seconds (SEE FIGURE 13-5). Lastly, bring the legs to 30° (SEE FIGURE 13-6). Maintain the stretch of the arms and the strong leg action. Hold the pose for several breaths.

FIGURE 13-6:
Legs at 30
degrees

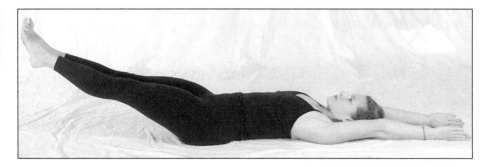

Exhale and smoothly lower the legs to the ground with control. Bring the arms to the side and relax (SEE FIGURE 13-7). To repeat, bend the legs to bring the legs up to 90°.

FIGURE 13-7:
End of pose

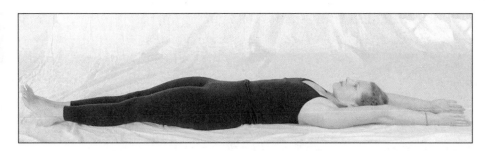

You can also practise this pose by placing the palms under the buttocks throughout the pose for support of the lower back. If you have difficulty with the pose, begin practising with one leg raised at a time until the back and abdomen become stronger and endurance improves. You can also try keeping one leg bent, with the foot on the floor, while the other leg is raised and lowered.

If you feel lower back pain throughout the pose and its variations, don't do the pose. The pose is also not recommended during pregnancy or menstruation.

The benefits of Urdhva Prasarita Padasana include the following:

· It strengthens abdominal muscles.
· It strengthens lower back muscles.
· It improves digestion.
· It reduces fat around the abdomen.

ANANTASANA

Anantasana is the serpent pose. Lie on the back and roll onto the left side. Stack the left and right hips, knees and ankles over one another. Reach your left arm along the floor and bend it, allowing your palm to support your head at the base of the skull (feel the skull lengthen away from the neck, providing a nice stretch). Ground the outside of the left arm.

Lengthen through the left side of the body all the way to the feet. Stretch the heels away from the legs and lift the arches. Inhale and bend the right leg, with the knee facing the ceiling. The knee will want to come forward and the top hip will want to drop back. Try to maintain the stacking action of the hips by firming the top buttock forwards. Bring the right arm in front of the right leg and grasp the big toe or outside of the foot. Exhale and extend the right leg up. Have the inner right leg face forwards (SEE FIGURE 13-8). Gaze straight ahead.

FIGURE 13-8:
Anantasana

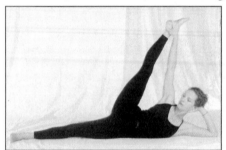

Lengthen from the back of both legs to the heels, firm the kneecaps and the front thighs. Maintain the extension of the front of the body, from the hips to the armpits. Hold the pose for several breaths, and then release and change sides.

You can also practise this pose by pressing both feet into the wall to get maximum stretch in the legs. Keep the bottom foot actively pressing into the wall as you raise the top leg. Or, instead of raising the upper leg, place it in front of the lower leg, with the foot on the floor facing the straight leg foot (SEE FIGURE 13-9). Press the foot down and feel the groin stretch. You can also try using a belt around the raised foot of the upward-extended leg to create more ease in the pose (SEE FIGURE 13-10).

FIGURE 13-9:
Anantasana,
with front leg
bent and foot
on floor

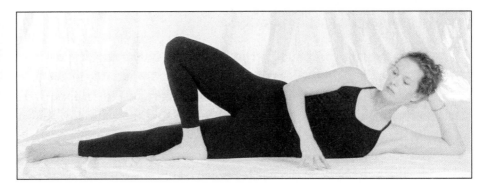

FIGURE 13-10:
Anantasana
with belt

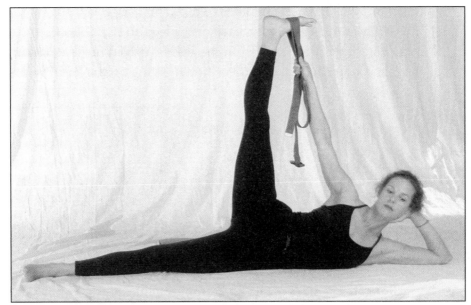

The benefits of Anantasana include the following:

· It relieves backache.
· It stretches and tones the hamstrings.
· It's healthy for the pelvic organs.

SUPTA PADANGUSTHASANA I

Supta Padangusthasana I is the reclining-hand-on-the-big-toe pose. Lie down and extend the legs on the floor. Stretching into the feet, lengthen into the crown of the head. Bend the right leg and extend it up to perpendicular, with the sole of the foot facing the ceiling. Hold onto the big toe with the first two fingers, or hold onto the outside of the foot (SEE FIGURE 13-11).

Press the back of the left leg down. Fully stretch both legs in two directions, knee to heel and knee to hip. This action will extend the legs more fully and help keep the back of the legs on the floor. Lengthen the inner and outer heels away from the ankles, spread the toes and lift the inner and outer arches. Feel the action drawing up the legs.

FIGURE 13-11:
Supta
Padangusth-
asana, begin-
ning pose

FIGURE 13-12:
With belt

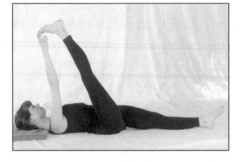 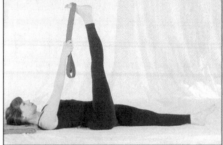

Elongate the sides of the body from the hips to the armpits. Lengthen from the right waist to the hip to equalize both sides of the body. The right side will want to shorten due to the leg being raised. Avoid this by maintaining the length on both sides of the body. Stay in the pose for several breaths, and then lower the leg and repeat on the other side.

You can also practise this pose using a belt around the balls of the outstretched foot. Hold on to each side of the strap with each hand (SEE FIGURE 13-12). To make the pose more comfortable for your hamstrings, bend the bottom leg, with your foot flat on the floor (SEE FIGURE 13-13). You can also slightly bend the upper leg (SEE FIGURE 13-14). Try placing the bottom foot against a wall for enhanced stretching of the bottom leg.

FIGURE 13-13:
With belt and
one leg bent

FIGURE 13-14:
With belt and
both legs bent

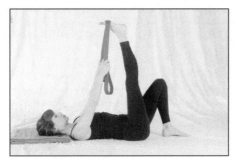 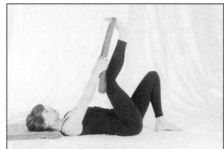

This pose isn't suitable for pregnant women. If you're pregnant, you can do the same pose while standing against the wall (refer to Hasta Padangusthasana I, p 105).

The benefits of Supta Padangusthasana I include the following:

· It develops the leg muscles.
· It balances the action of the leg muscles, so they work synergistically with each other.
· It lengthens the back muscles and hamstring muscles.
· It relieves sciatica.
· It increases hip flexibility and strength.
· It's excellent for health of the reproductive organs and provides relief from menstrual pain.

SUPTA PADANGUSTHASANA II

Lie down and raise the right leg to perpendicular. Grasp the big toe or hold onto the outside of the foot. Fully stretch the legs throughout the pose. On an exhalation, lower the right leg down to the right side (SEE FIGURE 13-15, p172). The hips must remain level with each other, so the leg may not reach the floor. Look at the ceiling. Remain in the pose for a few breaths and then carefully raise the leg back up to perpendicular, release the grasp of the hand and lower the leg to the floor. Repeat on the other side.

You can also practise this pose by placing a belt around the outstretched leg and hold onto the strap with the same hand as the raised leg (SEE FIGURE 13-16). Bend the bottom leg, foot flat on the floor, to make it more comfortable for the hamstrings. Place the bottom foot against a wall for enhanced stretching of the bottom leg.

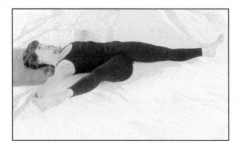
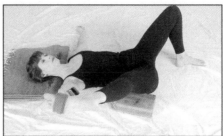

FIGURE 13-15:
Beginning pose

FIGURE 13-16:
With belt, support under the thigh, and a bent leg

This pose is not suitable for pregnant women. If you're pregnant, you can do the same pose while standing against the wall (see Hasta Padangusthasana II, p 285).

The benefits of Supta Padangusthasana II include the following:

- It develops the leg muscles.
- It balances the action of the leg muscles, so they work synergistically with each other.
- It lengthens the back muscles and hamstring muscles.
- It relieves sciatica.
- It increases hip flexibility and strength.
- It's excellent for health of the reproductive organs, and provides relief from menstrual pain.

CAT POSE

This pose warms up the spine beautifully, creating suppleness and strengthening the back muscles. Start on all fours, with your wrists under your shoulders and your knees under your hips. Look forward and lengthen into the crown of the head and into the coccyx. Inhale the breath. Slightly tip the coccyx up and lift the head (refer to FIGURE 9-18, p 90), without over-arching the back and dropping the waist (this will compress the lower back, resulting in pain). Broaden the buttock bones.

Exhale, pressing the hands and the tops of the feet down and away from the body as you round the spine by curling the chin into the chest and lifting each vertebra up toward the ceiling. Draw the coccyx in between the legs, towards the pubis bone (refer to FIGURE 9-19, p 91) as the pubis bone moves toward the navel and the navel recedes and presses up to the front of the spine. Repeat the lengthening on the inhalation and rounding on the exhalation nine more times, coordinating the movement with the breath.

Inhale and lengthen the spine. Exhale and draw the right knee and the chin into the chest while rounding the back. Repeat this pattern five times and then change sides. You can also try starting on all fours and shifting your weight onto your right hip. Inhale and lengthen the spine. Exhale and turn the head and the whole left side of the body to look at the right hip. With each successive exhalation, try to bring the head closer to the hip. This action will create stretch on the left side of the body and contraction on the right side of the body. As you inhale, feel the breath come into the left side, which has been stretched and opened to receive the breath. Once you've gone as far as you can go (without aggressive action), come back to the centre and repeat on the left side.

This variation has been called threading the needle: starting on all fours, thread your right arm under the body to the left side. Rest your right ear and the top of the right shoulder on the floor. The left arm is bent at a 90° angle and the palm is flat on the floor. Take several breaths in this position. If comfortable, place the left palm on the sacrum (the small of the back). This will increase the intensity of the pose somewhat, so go back if the first position is enough for you. With each exhalation, draw the left shoulder and elbow easily behind you. Stay for several breaths and then unthread the right arm and come back to table position. This is a twisting pose. Repeat on the other side.

Starting on all fours, inhale and lift and extend the right arm and the left leg. Exhale and stretch into the fingers and the toes. After a few breaths, come back into table position and then repeat with the opposite arm and leg. This variation helps strengthen the muscles of the back and the back of the leg while also creating extension.

The Cat Pose and its variations have the following benefits:

· They increase the flexibility and suppleness of the spine
  and its surrounding muscles.
· They work the entire spine.
· They stretch and tone the muscles of the back.
· They plump up the spinal discs and aid in fluid circulation in
  and out of the discs.
· They stimulate the nervous system.
· They're useful as a warm-up for other postures and as a way
  of stretching the back side of the body after backbending.
· They teach coordination of the breath with movement.
· They release tension in the back.

Yoga is great for children. Here are some of the benefits:

- It improves concentration and focus.
- It decreases stress and tension.
- It is calming and centring.
- It develops coordination.
- It develops agility and grace.
- It is playful, energizing and empowering.
- It improves self-esteem.
- It improves body image.
- It deepens a connection with self when peer pressure is strong.
- It balances emotions.

ADHO MUKHA SVANASANA

Adho Mukha Svanasana is the downward-facing dog pose. If you've ever
seen a dog stretching, you know that this pose looks like an upside-down
V. It is beautiful to watch. The dog grounds into his four paws and then
lengthens up the front legs and back legs, through the spine, to the

buttocks. It looks so easy and natural, and it is a terrific stretch! Downward-facing dog is one of the most frequently practised yoga poses.

Start on the hands and knees. Place the hands under the shoulders and the knees directly under the hips. The inner arms face each other, and the elbows are straight and firm (SEE FIGURE 13-17). Let the shoulder blades come onto the back. Observe that the upper arm bones connect into the shoulder socket. The pelvis is in a neutral position, horizontal to the floor. Tuck the toes under.

Plant the hands firmly on the floor and spread the fingers evenly apart. Press the palms, knuckles and fingers into the floor. Especially press down the index-finger knuckle and balance the weight on either side of the hand (just like you do for the feet in standing poses). These are important actions to maintain throughout the pose, because the hands are part of the pose's foundation, and they must stay rooted in order for extension of the spine to occur.

FIGURE 13-17:
Adho Mukha
Svanasana,
from all fours

FIGURE 13-18:
Adho Mukha
Svanasana

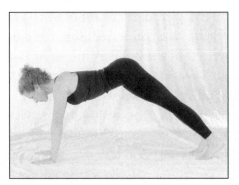
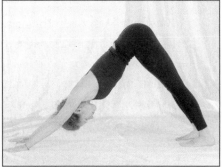

Inhale the breath, lift the hips evenly and press the hands and feet down (FIGURE 13-18). On the exhalation, straighten the legs and let the head drop between the arms. Relax the neck. Press the front of the thighs back to elongate the torso. Press the hands down, extending into the fingertips. Then stretch the arms away from the hand, all the way up to the buttock bones. Let the spine lengthen from the top of the head to the coccyx, into one long line of extension (SEE FIGURE 13-19, p 176).

FIGURE 13-19:
Lengthening up
of the side
body and spine

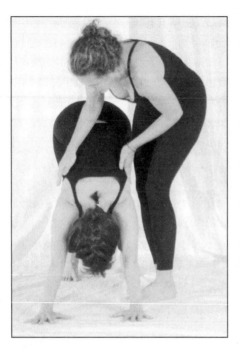

Lift the heels up, keeping the shoulders from moving forwards, and continue stretching all the way up the back of the legs to the buttock bones. Now lengthen the heels down, but keep stretching the back of the legs up. Lift the kneecaps and firm the thighs. The heels are stretching towards the floor. They might even make it to the floor, but do not force this action if it is not happening. Lift the shins out of the top of the ankles as you press the heels down. The feet are also working, spreading and grounding, with arches lifting to enhance the upward extension of the legs. Fully stretch the legs. Keep the arms as long as possible. Bending the elbows will make it difficult to transfer the weight of the body from the arms to the legs. Remain in the pose for several breaths, extending the spine on the inhalation. Then bend the knees and come down.

You can put the back of the heels against the wall for extra grounding. Or try placing the hands and feet wider apart than shoulder width. This helps ease tight shoulders and hips and is a good way to start practising downward-facing dog. If the hamstrings are tight, keep the knees slightly bent and focus on lengthening the spine and drawing the coccyx up and back. As time goes on and the hamstrings loosen, fully stretch the legs.

For a more challenging way to come into downward-facing dog, lie on your front, with your hands on the floor under the shoulders, and fingers facing forwards. Extend the legs behind you and tuck the toes under. Inhale the breath, press the hands and the toes down and stretch the arms up, lifting the body off the floor. The body is compact, with no sagging of the abdomen, hips and thighs. Lift the hips and buttocks up, bend the hips and press the legs back into downward-facing dog.

If you have wrist problems, you can put a rolled-up hand towel under the wrists to bring the weight into the knuckles and fingers and take pressure off the wrists. Practise with awareness, gradually building up strength in the hands and wrists.

If you have shoulder pain during Adho Mukha Svanasana, pay particular attention to how weight is distributed through the hands, arms and shoulders, and transferred up the spine to the coccyx. Of course, if there is pain, come down from the pose.

The benefits of Adho Mukha Svanasana include the following:

·   It stretches hamstring and calf muscles.
·   It lengthens and tractions the spine.
·   It strengthens the upper body, arms and wrists.
·   It's great for increasing bone density as a weight-bearing exercise.
·   It increases shoulder flexibility.
·   It opens the chest.
·   As a mild inversion, the heart is rested and the brain is quietened.

ARDHA MANDALASANA

Ardha Mandalasana is a lunge pose. Get onto all fours. Look forwards and bring the left leg forwards, planting the left foot between the hands. Place the fingertips alongside the left foot. Spread the toes and balls of the feet, and lift the arches. The left shin is perpendicular to the floor, with the knee over the heel.

Extend the right leg from the hip to the heel with the toes tucked under. Lift the back thigh away from the floor slightly, to ensure that the thigh bone is feeding into the socket, rather than hanging out of the socket (hanging from the hip joint is detrimental to the health of the joint and its surrounding ligaments and tendons). Ground the left foot and toes of the right foot.

Maintain the extension of the spine from the coccyx to the crown of the head. Press into the fingertips and stretch the arms up into the shoulder sockets to support the upper body (SEE FIGURE 13-20). Hold the pose for several breaths, then release and repeat on the left side.

FIGURE 13-20:
With extended
back leg

FIGURE 13-21:
With blocks
and extended
back leg

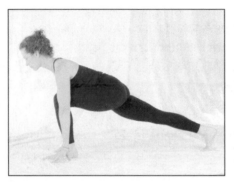 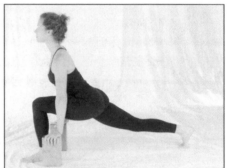

You can also try bending the back knee and resting it on the floor. This action will increase the opening and lengthening of the groin and the front of the back thigh. Place blocks at an appropriate height under the hands for comfort and to increase the pose and to maintain the length of the arms and the extension of the spine out of the pelvis (SEE FIGURE 13-21).

The benefits of Ardha Mandalasana include the following:

- It improves range of motion and flexibility of the hips.
- It stretches and opens the groin and the psoas muscle.
- It warms up and prepares the body for backbends by opening the groin.

RAJA KAPOTASANA MODIFIED

Raja Kapotasana Modified is the pigeon pose. Start on all fours. Bring the right leg through as in the lunge pose. Once the right foot is between the feet, let the right side of the leg rest on the floor. The outside of the right shin and thigh will be against the floor. Your fingertips will be on either side of the right leg. Adjust the angles of the right leg so there is some comfort in the posture. The further forward the shin is, the more intense the stretch will be on the right buttock, outer hip and outer thigh. It is fine to bring the right heel close in towards the pubis. Tuck the toes of the back leg under to provide more muscle energy in the back leg.

Observe how you are balanced in this pose. The tendency is to sit more onto the bent leg side. Try to balance your weight between the two legs by rolling more onto the straight (back) leg side.

Prop yourself up on your arms by placing the fingertips of each hand on the floor stretching up through the arms and the spine. Let the hips sink down as if you were sitting. Stretch into the back heel (SEE FIGURE 13-22). Stay for several breaths, then come back onto all fours and repeat on the other side.

Use blocks under the hands to help lift the spine and create more ease in the pose. You can also try bending forwards from the hips into a forward bend (SEE FIGURE 13-23). Extend the arms forward on the floor and rest the forehead on the floor, or fold the arms, hold onto the elbows and rest the forehead. As another modification, while in the forward bend position, try walking the hands to the right to increase the stretch on the left side of the body.

FIGURE 13-22:
Modified, with
blankets

FIGURE 13-23:
Modified, with
blankets, as for-
ward bend

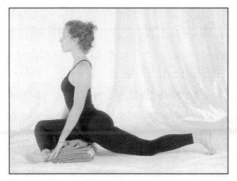
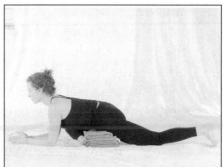

You can also fold two blankets into eighths and come into pigeon pose with the upper half of the right thigh and the buttock bone on the blanket. The shin will be on the floor in front of the blankets, and the left leg will be behind the blankets.

The benefits of the pigeon pose include the following:

· It stretches the piriformis muscle located between the hip and the sacrum (a tight piriformis muscle can cause sciatic nerve pain by pressing on the nerve as it leaves the sciatic notch).
· It opens and releases the external hip rotator muscles, which get tight from running, cycling and sitting.
· It stretches the iliotibial band on the outside of the thigh.
· It readjusts the sacrum.
· It stretches the psoas muscle in the groin.

BALASANA

Balasana is the child's pose. Start on all fours, with the hands under the shoulders and the knees under the hips. Inhale, and on the exhalation draw your buttocks back to rest on your heels. Press the hands on the floor, extending into the fingertips and stretching back through the sides of the body to the hips. Let the forehead rest on the floor (refer to FIGURE 9-20, p 91). While in the pose, inhale and feel the expansion of the waist and lower back. Exhale and observe the contraction of the ribs and lungs as the breath leaves the body. Stay for several breaths and then come back up and release the pose.

If the head does not reach the floor, place a folded blanket under the forehead. If the buttocks do not meet the heels, place a folded blanket between the heels and blanket for support. Walk the hands to the right for several breaths and then to the left. This stretches one side of the body at a time, and is particularly beneficial for scoliosis, where one side of the body is convex and the other is concave.

You can also try placing two blocks under the hands. Press down on the blocks actively, and lift the arms away from the floor. Observe how the upper arm feeds into the shoulder socket and the shoulder blades come onto the back. This is a good exercise to learn how the arms connect to the torso and how the shoulder blades hug the back.
It also develops upper-body strength.

For greater comfort, you can also place a blanket under the shins. If the knees are uncomfortable, place a folded blanket in the knee crease. As a restorative posture, place two to three vertically folded blankets under the torso, with the bent legs on either side of the support. Turn the head to one side for half the duration of the pose and then turn it the other way for the remaining time.

The benefits of Balasana include the following:

· It increases circulation in the lower back and abdomen.
· It stretches the back muscles and the spine.
· It eases lower back discomfort.
· It's a good resting pose to do between more strenuous postures.

PLANK POSE

Plank pose is a weight-bearing pose, which is good preparation for other poses emphasizing upper-body strength. Lie down on your front, bend your arms, and place the hands on the floor and under the shoulders (fingers facing forward). Extend the legs behind you and tuck the toes under (SEE FIGURE 13-24). The more you walk the toes toward the legs, the more activity and muscle-hugging bone action there will be in the legs.

FIGURE 13-24:
Preparation for
the
plank pose

FIGURE 13-25:
Plank pose

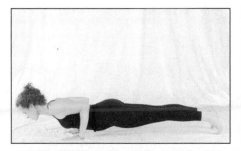
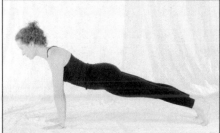

Press the hands down firmly and feel the upper back muscles start contracting and drawing into the shoulder blades and against the back. Now the actions of the hands, feet and legs have supplied the necessary support for the plank pose.

As you maintain these actions, press the hands and toes down, exhale into the lower abdomen and stretch the arms up into the shoulder sockets, lifting the torso and legs off the floor. Make sure the shoulder blades are supporting and opening the chest. Stretch the heels away from the body as the kneecaps and the front of the thighs firm and stretch toward the hips. The body, from the shoulders to the hips and feet, forms a slanted line of strength and alignment (SEE FIGURE 13-25, p 181). Hold the pose for several breaths and then come down.

As in downward-facing dog, you can place support under the wrist to distribute the weight into the knuckles and fingers. You can also try getting into plank pose from downward-facing dog. Bring the shoulders over the wrists and lower the hips, while stretching and firming the arms and legs and pulling the heels away from the legs. Be careful not to let the abdomen, hips and thighs sag, or the lower back will get compressed. If you have wrist pain, use support under the wrist. If pain persists, come out of the pose.

The benefits of the plank pose include the following:

· It increases upper-body strength.
· It develops upper-back muscles.
· It's an excellent weight-bearing exercise for increasing bone density.
· It opens the chest.

CHATTARANGA DANDASANA

FIGURE 13-26:
Chattaranga
Dandasana

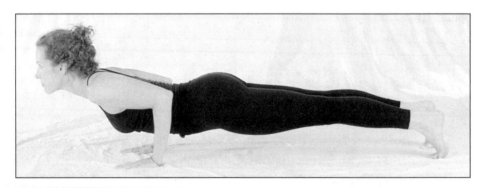

Chattaranga Dandasana is the four-limbed staff pose. In this pose, the body resembles a staff, parallel to the ground, which is supported by the strength of the four limbs. Lie down on your front with legs extended and hands under shoulders, fingers facing forward. The elbows are next to the waist, not out to the sides. Press the hands down and lift the top of the shoulders away from the floor. The goal is to have the shoulder at the same height as the elbows throughout the pose (SEE FIGURE 13-26). Otherwise, the upper arm bone will not be in the socket, and there is a possibility of injuring your neck and shoulders through misalignment. Observe the muscle action in the upper back. Feel the shoulder blades hugging the back.

Shrug the shoulders toward the ears slightly to feed the upper arm bones into the shoulder socket. Now the arms and shoulders are supporting the upper body. Tuck the toes under and walk them towards the body. This action helps lift the kneecaps and firms the thighs, drawing the muscle energy up the front of the leg to the hip. The thigh bones insert into the hip sockets, supporting the pelvis. Now stretch the heels away from the back body, stimulating muscle action through the back of the leg from hamstrings to heel. Feel the thighs and hips lift slightly off the floor.

Inhale, and as you exhale press the lower abdomen against the front of the spine, press the hands and toes down, and lift the body, like a staff, up off the floor. Lengthen the collarbones and sternum towards the head and the abdomen and lower back toward the heels. The hips and shoulders are the same height off the floor. See if you can stay up for a second and come down. Try it several times, using your breath to facilitate the movement into the pose.

Remember that in the *Yoga Sutra,* the importance of *sadhana* (practice) is stressed over and over, as an integral part of the path of yoga. Your strength and agility will improve over time, so don't be discouraged if it seems impossible at first.

As a modification, try getting into the pose from downward-facing dog. Bring the shoulders over the wrists and bend the arms back into Chattaranga Dandasana arms as you compactly lower your body parallel to the floor. Stretch your sternum forwards and your abdomen and heels away from the sternum. Press the soles of the feet against the wall to feel the action of the heels stretching backward.

This pose is not to be done by pregnant women once the stomach is protruding. People with wrist problems should do the pose carefully, using support under the wrist to decrease the angle of the bend in the wrist. Distribute the body weight through the entire hand, not just the wrist. Press the fingers down as you lengthen into the fingertips. If you have shoulder problems, check your alignment. Make sure the shoulders remain in line with the elbows. Hold the pose briefly and repeat several times, unless pain is present.

The benefits of Chattaranga Dandasana include the following:

- It increases upper-body strength.
- It increases bone density.
- It strengthens the arms and wrists.
- It improves wrist flexibility.
- It contracts and tones abdominal organs.

SPHINX POSE

Lie on your front with legs extended behind you. Prop yourself up on your forearms. Your forearms will be parallel to each other, with the elbows close to the waist and in line with the wrists and shoulders. Press the forearms and the palms down, and observe how this grounding action lifts the chest and elongates the sides of the body. Maintaining this action, pull the elbows back on the floor without actually moving them. Feel the muscles of the upper back draw into the back and hug the shoulder blades. Enhance this by lifting the sternum forwards and up. Enjoy the openness and broadness of the top chest. Stay for several breaths and then release down and rest (refer to FIGURE 9-15, p 88).

The benefits of the sphinx pose include the following:

- It strengthens the upper back muscles.
- It opens the chest and stretches the muscles on the front body.
- It teaches basic back-bending action.

BHUJANGASANA

Bhujangasana is the cobra pose. Lie on your front with your forehead on the floor, your hands under your shoulders and your legs outstretched together behind you. Press the hands and the front of the feet down and lengthen the toes away from the body. Draw the elbows into the waist.

Inhale and look forwards. Feel the breath ease as the chest opens. Stretch the chest, the area between the shoulder blades (upper back) and the ribs forward. The ribs and the stomach move away from the hips, and the hips stretch away from the legs. The pubic bone remains on the floor and the lower back and coccyx lengthen away from the upper body (SEE FIGURE 13-27). Space is created between the hips and the ribs, allowing the spine to lengthen into the body. The stomach receives a pleasant stretch. Make sure you exhale completely.

Coil the spine into the body like a wave that is moving in and up to arc before it spills over into the surf. Use your hands, pressing down to lengthen the arms up to support the coiling action of the spine. The arms do not have to straighten, and they should not be used to create a pushing-up feeling (which will cause shortening of the lower back and compression). Breathe! Do not hold breath in.

FIGURE 13-27:
Bhujangasana

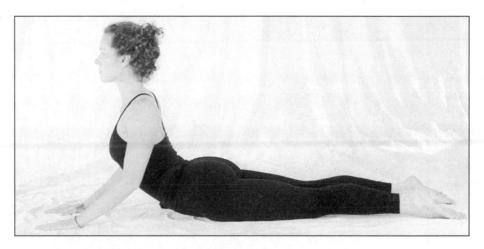

Come up only as far as is comfortable for you. If there is lower back discomfort, you have come up too far through the pushing-up action of the arms. The arms are there only to provide extra support. Stay in the pose for a few breaths and then come down. Repeat several times, going up and coming down.

As you coil the spine in and up, you can also try letting the hands come off the floor. Continue lengthening the upper back, chest and ribs forwards and up. Practising in this way will allow the upper back muscles to strengthen and draw in to support the spine and upper body. Without the use of the hands and arms, the lower back will remain spacious and long (SEE FIGURE 13-28).

FIGURE 13-28:
Bhujangasana
modified, with
hands hovering
over floor,
emphasizing
coiling of spine

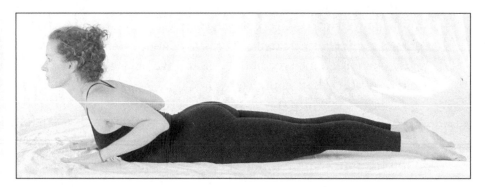

Try placing a folded blanket under the lower belly and hips (SEE FIGURE 13-29). Do the pose. The elevation of the lower abdomen and hips lessens the risk of lower-back compression.

FIGURE 13-29:
Bhujangasana
modified, with
blankets under
pelvis and
hands forward
of shoulders

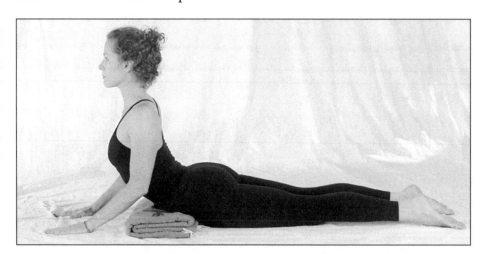

This pose is not recommended for pregnant women. If you have lower back pain, practise the pose non-aggressively.

The benefits of Bhujangasana include the following:

· It stretches the front side of the body and its organs.
· It strengthens the spine and back muscles and relieves backache.
· It squeezes, tones and stimulates organs in the back of the body.
· When done correctly, it can relieve sciatica and slipped disc (**best done under the supervision of a qualified yoga professional**).

The coiling, wavelike action of the spine drawing in and up creates the backbend and the space between the vertebrae necessary for a safe backbend. The entire spine must be involved in stretching, or pain will be felt in the weaker parts of the back.

URDHVA MUKHA SVANASANA

Urdhva Mukha Svanasana is the upward-facing dog pose – the counter-pose to downward-facing dog. It is a backbend, while downward-facing dog is a forward bend. Urdhva Mukha Svanasana has similar actions to the cobra pose, the difference being that the legs come off the floor in upward-facing dog.

Lie down on your front. Extend the legs straight out behind you. Place your hands by your waist, fingers facing forward. Stretch from the legs to the toes and hug the thigh muscle into the bone. Inhale and look forwards. Extend your chest and your upper back forward and your ribs forwards and up. Draw the ribs away from the stomach to create space for the spine to come in, lengthen, and coil.

Press the hands and feet down to lift the legs slightly off the floor and to support the torso. Exhale. Stretch into the toes as you continue coiling the spine forwards and up. Bring the upper arms back and open the top chest to draw the shoulder blades into the back. Lift the kneecaps and firm the thighs. Avoid over-squeezing the shoulder blades together, creating a crease between them. The shoulder blades move into the back body. Gaze upwards if the neck is comfortable, or else look forwards. Feel the stretch in the stomach. Stay in the pose for several natural, smooth breaths, and then come down and release.

You can also tuck the toes under instead of coming up on the front of the feet (SEE FIGURE 13-30). This will stimulate muscle-hugging action in the legs. When using the arms in the pose, bend the elbows out to the sides and press the chest and upper back forwards. Then lengthen the arms. Do this several times. This enhances the expansion of the chest and the drawing in of the shoulder blades against the back. You may also want to try doing the pose while keeping the knees on the floor (SEE FIGURE 13-31).

If you have wrist problems, use support under the wrist to change the angle of flexing. Distribute the weight evenly throughout the hand. If you have lower back pain, don't push aggressively into the pose. Create as much space as possible in the spine. Draw the ribs forward and lengthen the sacrum and coccyx down and away from the lower back. Often the thighs lift too high off the ground, causing the lower back to pop up and shorten and compress. The thighs lift only in reaction to the pressing down of the feet.

FIGURE 13-30:
With toes
tucked under

FIGURE 13-31:
With knees on
floor, toes
tucked under

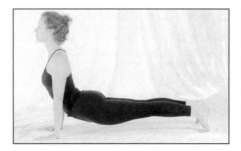 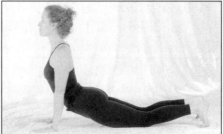

The benefits of Urdhva Mukha Svanasana include the following:

- It is a wonderful stretch in the front body and its organs.
- It is excellent for flexibility of the spine.
- It strengthens back muscles and the spine.
- It increases bone density.
- It relieves backache such as sciatica and slipped disc.
- It expands the chest and increases lung capacity.
- It improves circulation in the pelvis.

SALABHASANA

Salabhasana is the locust pose. This is another prone backbend, which gradually arches the back. Lie on the front, with the legs together and extended. Stretch into the toes. Reach the arms out in front on the floor, with the palms facing each other. Stretch into the fingertips. Inhale, and exhale as you firm your abdominals. Keeping the abdominals firm, inhale, lift and extend the arms and legs. Keep breathing and lengthening into the fingers and toes. Think of lengthening your front body without shortening your back body. The head should be between the arms and at arm height (SEE FIGURE 13-32). If the head is higher than the arms, the back of the neck will be shortened. After several breaths, exhale and release the pose. Rest on your front with your head to the side. Repeat two more times.

FIGURE 13-32:
Salabhasana

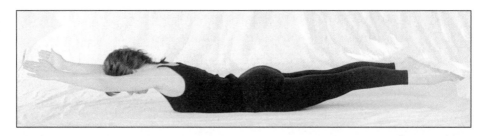

You can also start Salabhasana more gradually to build up strength and stamina. First, inhale and lift the right arm (SEE FIGURE 13-33). Next, lift the right arm with the left leg, and then raise the left arm with the right leg (SEE FIGURE 13-34, p 190). The arms and legs can be raised separately. Last, raise the same arm with same leg. Remember to lengthen and lift for extension, not for height or contraction of the lower back muscles.

FIGURE 13-33:
Salabhasana
with single arm
raised, head in
line with arm

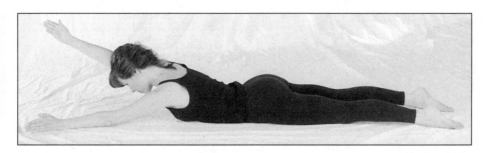

You can also change the arm position. Bring the arms out to the side or clasped behind you, holding onto a belt. Stretch the chest up, and draw the shoulder blades into the back of the body.

FIGURE 13-34:
Salabhasana
with alternate
arm and leg
raised, head in
line with arm

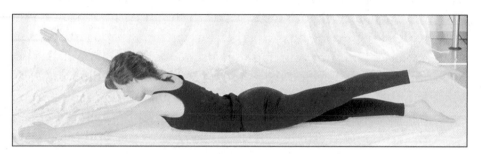

The benefits of Salabhasana include the following:

· It creates a long curve of the spine.
· It strengthens the entire back of the body.
· It stimulates the spleen and the pancreas.

CHAPTER 14

Inverted Postures and Balance Poses

nverted postures reverse the effects of gravity. Everything is turned upside down. The head, hands or forearms are now the base of the poses, while the legs and feet lengthen up to the sky. Balance poses develop coordination, poise, agility and grace, increasing strength and stamina. Focus and concentration improve. *Pratyahara*, withdrawal of the senses, is practised, as you must go deep inside and become quiet to balance.

SALAMBA SARVANGASANA FOR BEGINNERS

Salamba Sarvangasana is a shoulderstand. Stack three folded blankets on top of each other, rounded edges together and facing away from the wall, 30cm (12in) or so away from the wall. The top edge of the blankets is rounded (this is where the blanket was folded) and firmer than the bottom edge of the blankets. Lie down on the blankets, with the head and neck off the top, rounded edge of the blankets. There should be 2.5cm or more of space between the shoulders and the top edge of the blankets, so when you roll onto the top of the shoulders, the shoulders do not roll onto the floor. Your knees are bent with your feet on the wall at a 90° angle (adjust your distance to the wall so the legs can be at 90°). The buttocks are on the floor. Have your arms by your sides and roll the upper arms out, so the palms are facing up.

Bend the elbows and press the upper arms down, and as you inhale lift the buttocks up. Support the lower back with the hands (SEE FIGURE 14-1). The head is on the floor, the shoulders are on the blankets, but the neck will be slightly off the floor. This is important for the health of the neck and for retaining its natural curve. If the neck pressed down onto the floor, this could be injurious to the neck and could, in time and with repeated practice, cause a flattening of the natural curve of the cervical spine. Then the pose would be a neckstand rather than a shoulderstand.

FIGURE 14-1:
Sarvangasana with bent legs and feet on the wall

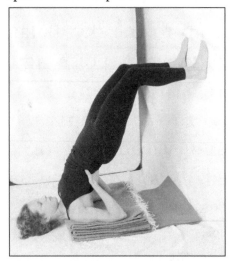

Lifting the buttocks off the floor causes you to roll onto the top of the shoulders. The foundation in shoulderstand is the top of the shoulders and the upper arms. The upper arms press down, to allow the body and legs to extend up. The shoulder blades press into the back, opening the chest and drawing the upper spine into the body. The hands support the torso, but it is the back muscles and the lifting of the legs out of the pelvis that work to hold you up in shoulderstand. Try to keep the elbows shoulder-width apart and under the shoulders for alignment and support. (Tight shoulders will make it difficult to bring the elbows to shoulder width.) As you remain in the pose, see if you can move the hands down toward the shoulder blades every few breaths.

Stay for several breaths, keeping the throat soft, then release the hands from the back and slowly lower to the ground. After practising this variation of shoulderstand for several weeks, start extending one leg at a time, straight up, stretching up through the leg to the heel. Then, when you feel ready, try raising both legs off the wall, and press down through the upper arms, as you lift up through the ribs, lower back and legs. Bring the legs back to the wall and come down.

When you have come down from shoulderstand, it is a good idea to rest the back muscles, which have worked hard to hold you up in the posture. With knees bent and feet flat on the floor, move in the direction of your head so the waist is on the top edge of the blankets, where the shoulders were in the pose. Keep the knees bent and the feet on the floor. The arms are off the blankets with the palms facing up. After several breaths, move the body further toward the head until the buttocks are off the blankets. The knees are still bent and the feet are on the floor. Rest and let the back muscles soften and release. Cross the legs at the ankles and let the thighs rest on the blankets. Rest for several breaths. Then change the cross of the legs. After a few breaths, uncross the legs, roll onto the right side and slowly come up to a seated position.

It is important not to turn the head while in shoulderstand, as this could be injurious to the neck. The throat should remain soft throughout the posture.

You can also practice Sarvangasana by placing a belt looped to shoulder width around the right elbow and then lying down with the head and neck off the blankets and the shoulders on the blankets. Do not try this variation the first time you try to do Sarvangasana. When you bring the legs over the head, place the other end of the belt loop around your left elbow behind your back, and then extend the legs up. Using a belt does not allow the elbows to splay apart wider than the width of your shoulders, providing alignment and support.

Try placing a chair behind the blankets, with the chair seat facing the blankets. Lie down on the blankets and extend the arms over your head, holding onto the chair legs with your hands. This is the correct distance for the chair to be away from the body. Bring the arms back to the sides of the body and bend the knees, feet flat on the floor. Inhale, bend the knees to the chest, press and firm the upper arm bones down onto the blankets for foundation, and swing the hips and legs over the head. Place the tips of the toes on the chair seat.

FIGURE 14-2:
Ardha
Halasana with
chair and belt

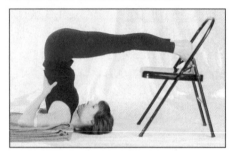

Support your back with your hands and adjust your arms, if necessary. Press the tips of the toes down on the chair seat to firm and lift the thighs up. Walk the toes back so you are resting on the top of the shoulders, not the shoulder blades. Tuck your shoulders under and roll the upper arm bones under (SEE FIGURE 14-2). Now stretch your right leg up to 90° while the lower leg also stretches. Then bring the right leg down and extend the left leg up. Do this several times. (SEE FIGURE 14-3.) Next lift one leg up and then the other into shoulderstand. Hold for several breaths. Lower one leg down at a time to the chair, pressing the tips of the toes down to maintain active legs. When both legs are on the chair, release the arms from the back and slowly lower the spine and legs to the floor.

FIGURE 14-3:
Eka Pada
Sarvangasana

FIGURE 14-4:
Coming
into
Sarvangasana

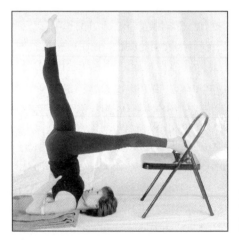
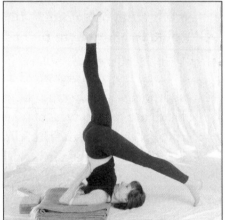

Instead of using the chair behind you, the tips of the toes can come onto the floor and then the legs can go up one at a time, into shoulder-stand. This requires flexibility in the lower back and the hamstrings. Once the back is strong, you can come right up into shoulderstand from the floor, one straight leg at a time (SEE FIGURES 14-4 AND 14-5).

FIGURE 14-5:
Sarvangasana
final pose

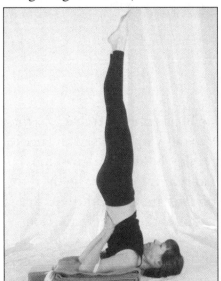

If you have neck problems, such as cervical spondylosis, work under the guidance of a qualified yoga professional. Do not hold the pose if the neck or shoulders hurt. This pose is not to be practised during menstruation, and it should not be performed by those people with heart problems, detached retina, ear problems or high blood pressure.

Shoulderstand is called the Queen of Yoga postures because of its myriad benefits.

The benefits of Salamba Sarvangasana include the following:

· It stimulates the thyroid and parathyroid glands.
· It increases blood flow to the heart and brain without strain.
· It opens the lungs for easier breathing.
· It is beneficial for those with palpitations, breathlessness, asthma, bronchitis and throat discomfort.
· It soothes and quietens the nervous system.
· It relieves fatigue.
· It boosts the functioning of the immune system.
· It improves sleep quality.
· It decreases insomnia.
· It improves digestion and elimination.
· It's good for functioning of the reproductive organs.
· It regulates menstrual flow.

Don't stay in a shoulderstand if there is pressure in the head, eyes, ears, or throat. Come out of the pose, readjust your position and the support under you, and then carefully get into the pose. If there is still pressure, come down and don't practise the pose for a while. Downward-facing dog and forward bends can be practised instead.

HALASANA

Halasana is the plough pose. Set up blankets as instructed for the shoulderstand. Lie down on the blankets with the head and neck off the top edge of the blankets and the shoulder 2.5cm or more away from the blanket edge. With knees bent and feet on the floor, press the upper arm bones down and lift and swing the hips up as the legs go over the head. Press the tips of the toes into the floor and stretch into the heels.

Lift the front of the thigh to the back of the thigh, stretching the legs fully. Support the back with the hands (SEE FIGURE 14-6). Hold for several breaths, depending upon your comfort level and steadiness. Walk the hands down toward the shoulder blades every few breaths.

FIGURE 14-6:
Halasana

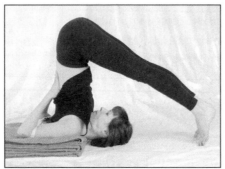

To come out of the pose, release the hands from the back and press the upper arms down as you slowly roll out of the pose. Bend the knees, feet flat on the floor, and move your body off the blankets toward your head, so the waist is on the top edge of the blankets where the shoulders were during the pose. After a few breaths resting in this position, move the buttocks off the blanket onto the floor and rest here for several breaths. Then cross the legs on the blanket and rest and change the cross and rest. Uncross the legs, roll onto the right side and press the hands down to bring yourself up to a seated position.

Sarvangasana (shoulderstand) and Halasana (plough pose) are usually done together. Try practising them this way, getting into Halasana first to set up the shoulders and arms properly for Sarvangasana. Then, after several breaths, get up into Sarvangasana, staying as long as you are comfortable and can maintain the extension of the spine and the lift and lengthening of the legs. Then, come back down into Halasana. Stay in Halasana according to your comfort and ease, and then come down and do the resting sequence described in Sarvangasana and Halasana.

If your feet don't reach the floor in Halasana, place a chair behind the blankets. Come into Halasana and place the tips of the toes on the chair seat (refer to FIGURE 14-2, p 194). Support the back with the hands. Observe whether you are on the top of the shoulders. Hold the pose, and when ready to come out, release the hands from the back, pressing the upper arm bones down and rolling out of the pose.

FIGURE 14-7:
Supported
Ardha
Halasana with
bent legs and
shins resting
on chair back

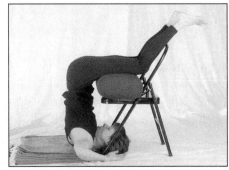

Halasana can be done as a passive, restorative pose by using a chair with a bolster or stack of folded blankets on the chair seat. The chair can be turned sideways if there is not enough room for the legs to go through the space between the chair back and the chair seat. As you get into the pose, the thighs rest on the bolster or blankets. The hands can support the back, or the arms can come out to the sides by the shoulders, with the elbows bent (SEE FIGURE 14-7).

If you suffer from ischemia or cervical spondylosis, do not perform Halasana. If you're subject to migraines, asthma or other breathing problems, high blood pressure, or fatigue, or if you're overweight, practise using props and with your eyes closed.

The benefits of Halasana include the following:

· It relieves fatigue.
· It improves digestion.
· It lengthens the back muscles and the spine, improving its alignment.
· It tones, squeezes and stimulates the abdominal organs.

- When done actively, not passively as a restorative pose, it strengthens the spine and the spinal muscles.
- In the rounded, restorative Halasana, the back muscles are lengthened.
- It helps relieve backache.
- It improves forward-bending ability by increasing suppleness of the back muscles and the hinging of the hip joint.

The arm, neck and back muscles and the spine must become stronger in order to maintain the shoulderstand and headstand postures. Begin daily (except during menstruation) with 30 seconds or 10 breaths in each pose. After two weeks of solid, safe practice, increase it to one minute. Thereafter, increase your time by 10 complete breaths or 30 seconds each month.

SETU BANDHASANA SARVANGASANA

Setu Bandhasana Sarvangasana, the bridge pose, is a restorative pose that provides similar benefits to shoulderstand. In fact, it is a good neck and upper body preparation for shoulderstand, as it stretches the neck and opens the chest, stretching the often tight upper chest muscles. Setu Bandhasana Sarvangasana can also be substituted for shoulderstand during menstruation.

Place two bolsters vertically one behind the other (or use four to six blankets vertically folded) on the floor. Lie with the whole body and legs on the bolsters, so the bottom edge of the shoulder blades are on the upper edge of the bolster. Loop a belt firmly around the middle of the thighs, so they will not be able to roll apart. An extra belt can also be looped around the middle of the shins for extra support.

The tops of the shoulders roll down to the floor, making a dome of, and expanding the upper chest. The back of the head is on the floor. The arms can be diagonally by your sides, with the palms facing up, or they can be bent at the elbows, like a cactus. The elbows will be in line with the shoulders (SEE FIGURE 14-8). Close the eyes and relax. Remain in the pose from 5 to 15 minutes. To come out of the pose, bend the knees with feet flat on the floor, and release the belt. Carefully move towards your head and bring your entire back and buttocks onto the floor, with knees bent. Then roll onto the right side and, using the hands, bring yourself up to a seated position.

FIGURE 14-8:
Setu
Bandhasana
supported

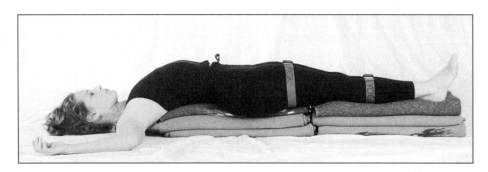

You can also practise this pose by raising the legs up higher to ease the back, or lowering the support under the torso for back comfort, or raising the support to increase the intensity of the pose (if appropriate). Pressing the feet into a wall will increase the stretch in the legs and the groin. You can place a rolled blanket under the neck for support, to encourage and maintain the natural curve of the neck. This is beneficial for those whose cervical spine has flattened.

The benefits of Setu Bandhasana Sarvangasana include the following:

·　It opens the chest and expands the lungs.
·　It improves quality and volume of the breath.
·　It stretches the front of the body.
·　It lengthens the groin and stretches the psoas muscles.
·　It calms and quietens the brain.
·　It soothes the nervous system.
·　It relieves backache.
·　It increases blood circulation to the arteries.
·　It decreases insomnia and stress headaches.
·　It improves digestion.
·　It rests the legs.
·　It prevents varicose veins.

Inverted postures should not be practised during menstruation, as they reverse the blood flow and could, potentially, disrupt the natural flow and cause abdominal discomfort. The only inversion recommended for people with high blood pressure, heart problems, detached retina and hearing problems is the legs-up-the-wall pose. Those with neck injuries must seek guidance from qualified yoga teachers about how to do inverted postures.

SIRSASANA

Sirsasana is the headstand. It is advisable to begin practising headstand after shoulderstand has become comfortable and can be held for at least eight minutes. Adho Mukha Svanasana (downward-facing dog) and Prasarita Padottanasana are also good preparation for Sirsasana. Initially, doing the headstand against a wall is recommended, until balance and upper-body strength are developed. Then you can start moving away from the wall little by little, to the centre of the room.

Place a folded blanket on the floor. Kneel and interlock the fingers (without gripping the fingers tight), with the cupped palms and forearms on the blanket. Start with the fingers as close to the wall as possible (still being able to come up into headstand). The elbows are no wider than the shoulders. Press the bottom of the wrists and the forearms strongly down on the blanket for foundation and grounding. Keep the shoulder blades on the back.

Place the crown of the head on the floor. The palms and interlocked fingers lightly cradle the back of the head. The little fingers touch the back of the head (not under it). Keep the neck extended. Tuck the toes under, inhale and lift the heels, hips and buttocks up, lengthening the spine from the crown of the head to the coccyx (SEE FIGURE 14-9). Stretch up through the back of the legs from the heels to the buttock bones. Lift the kneecaps and firm the front thighs up. These actions are much like downward-facing dog.

FIGURE 14-9:
Preparation for
Sirsasana

FIGURE 14-10:
Coming into
Sirsasana

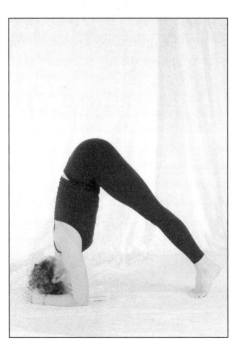

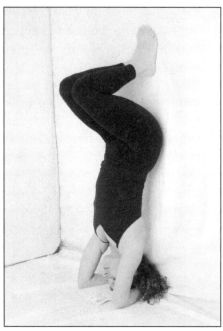

Now walk the feet in toward the torso as much as possible, while maintaining the length of the spine and the stretching of the legs. Bend the knees and lift the feet up, taking a small hop toward the buttocks and onto the wall (SEE FIGURE 14-10). The hips and balls of the feet rest on the wall.

Keep grounding the wrists and forearms. Firm the shoulder blades onto the back and lift them up. Lift the shoulders away from the ears. Let the weight of the head come into the floor as you lift the spine and the inner legs up. This two-way action of grounding the head and extending the spine and legs away from the head is crucial for developing space in the spine, rather than compression in the neck. Draw the shoulders away from the ears, and the shoulder blades up the back toward the kidneys.

Slowly lengthen the legs up. The back of the heels, hips and legs will touch the wall (SEE FIGURE 14-11, p 202). Stretch the heels up, lengthening the back of the legs away from the body, and press the balls of the feet up, elongating the front side of the legs. Lengthen the inner thighs to the inner heel to elongate and lift the core of the body up. Broaden the balls and heels of the feet. Lengthen the sides of the body, from the armpits to the soles of the feet. Gaze straight ahead. Hold the pose for several breaths.

FIGURE 14-11:
Sirsasana on
the wall

FIGURE 14-12:
Coming down
from Sirsasana

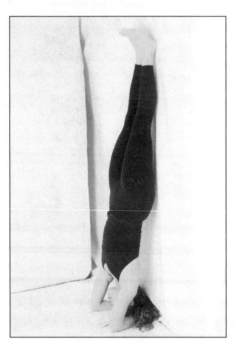 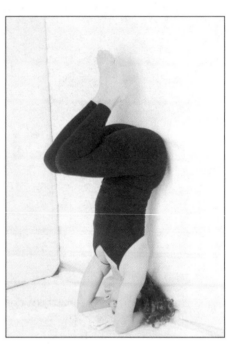

To come down, bend the knees while keeping the feet active. Slowly lower the legs as you draw the abdomen and groin up (SEE FIGURE 14-12). Bend the knees into the chest and let the feet come down to the floor. Rest in Balasana (child's pose) for a few breaths. It is important not to come up too quickly from an inversion, as dizziness and light-headedness can occur as a result of everything in the body having been upside down. Make a gradual transition back to your normal head-upright posture.

Before attempting headstand, practise headstand preparation: go up with interlocked fingers cradling the back of the head, and forearms on the ground (like downward-facing dog). Walk the legs in, maintain the

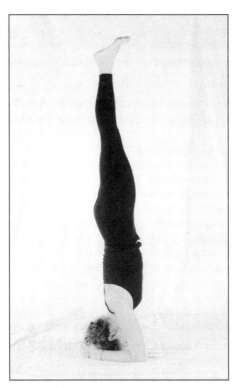

FIGURE 14-13:
Sirsasana

height in the spine and legs, and then bend the knees and come down into Balasana. Do this several times to get accustomed to having weight on the head and forearms. In time, with practice, bring the hips away from the wall, stretch up through the legs and learn to balance on your head, with the arms providing support (SEE FIGURE 14-13).

Sirsasana should not be practised during menstruation or by those with high blood pressure, detached retina, ear problems or cardiac disorders. Those people who have neck problems should practise under the supervision of a qualified yoga professional.

The benefits of Sirsasana include the following:

- It increases blood flow to the brain.
- It decreases fatigue.
- It enhances clarity of thought and concentration.
- It rests the heart.
- It stimulates the pituitary and pineal glands, which govern the body's health and growth.
- It strengthens the lungs.
- It increases resistance to colds, coughs and palpitations.
- It improves digestion and elimination.
- It decreases insomnia.
- It increases stamina and endurance.

Sirsasana (headstand) should always be followed by *Sarvangasana* (shoulderstand), even though shoulderstand is learned before headstand and can be practised without it. Headstand strengthens the neck; shoulderstand lengthens the neck. Any possibility of neck compression during headstand is countered by shoulderstand. Headstand without shoulderstand can make you irritable. Shoulderstand is soothing and balancing to the emotions.

VIPARITA KARANI

FIGURE 14-14:
Viparita Karani

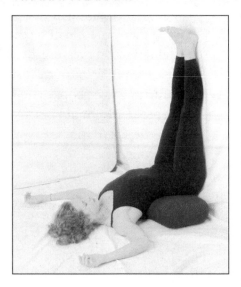

Viparita Karani is the legs-up-the-wall pose with support. Place a bolster or one to three horizontally folded blankets against a wall. Lie on your side with the left hip on the support, buttocks close to the wall and knees bent. Roll onto your back and swing the legs up the wall. Rest the legs on the wall, the lower back and sacrum on the support, and the rest of the torso on the floor (SEE FIGURE 14-14). Stretch the arms out horizontally with the palms facing up. The eyes may close and soften.

Breathe naturally and enjoy the relaxation and revitalization of the pose. To come out of the pose, bend the knees. With your feet on the wall, press yourself into the centre of the room with your knees bent and back resting on the floor. Then roll over onto your right side. Using your hands, press yourself up to a seated position.

You can also practise Viparita Karani with your legs separated wide apart. Alternatively, you can bend your knees slightly if it is too intense a stretch for the hamstring muscles.

Inversions are not recommended during menstruation. People with high blood pressure, hypertension, glaucoma and cardiac disorders should practise this posture **only** under the guidance of a qualified yoga professional. It is not advised for those people with detached retina and ear problems.

The benefits of Viparita Karani include the following:

· It drains fluid from the legs.
· It softens the stomach and groin.
· It reverses the effects of gravity.
· It reverses the flow of blood and lymph.
· It rests the heart and the brain.
· It relieves tired legs.
· It revitalizes and relaxes.

In inverted postures, there is increased blood and oxygen flow to the brain. The nervous system is strengthened, the heart rate slows and breathing deepens. Gravitational pressure on the abdominal organs is relieved while the diaphragm muscle rests on the lungs, toning and stimulating them. Organs are put back in their proper place after being pulled down by gravity.

VRKSASANA

Vrksasana, the tree pose, develops balance and upwards stretch, much like a tree, which has a strong, extensive root system, allowing it to grow tall and branch out.

Start by standing in Tadasana, or mountain pose. Gaze straight ahead with a soft but focused gaze. Shift your weight to the left leg, root down, spread the balls of the feet, broaden the heels and press firmly down with the big toe and little toe balls of the feet and the centre of each heel. Turn your right foot out to the side. Then bring your right foot up to the inside of the left leg to where it is comfortable. You can use your hand to help bring the foot up the leg. Press the sole of the right foot against the inside of the left leg, leg against foot, as if they were pressing the spine up. If the foot does not easily stay on the leg, it is fine to leave it on the floor turned out, with the right heel resting against the inner heel of the left foot. Maintain the grounding in the left foot and the extension in the left leg, taking care not to hyperextend the leg. Press the neck of the big toe down and lift the kneecap. Extend the arms out to the sides, with the palms facing up. Stretch all the way from the centre line in the body to the fingertips. On an inhalation, take the arms up over the head, stretching from the side ribs to the fingertips, palms facing each other (SEE FIGURE 14-15).

FIGURE 14-15:
Vrksasana

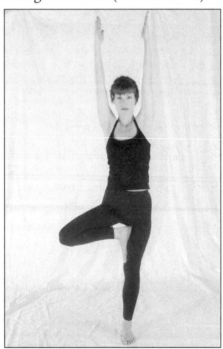

Continue breathing through the nostrils, relaxing the throat and diaphragm and softening the front ribs and stomach. Balance ease and effort. Stay in Vrksasana for several breaths, or as long as you feel comfortable and can maintain the pose. To come out of the pose, exhale and release the arms to the side as the right leg comes back into Tadasana. Repeat on the other side.

You can also practice Vrksasana with your arms wider apart, in the shape of a V, to maintain stretch and extension in the arms and straight elbows with which to lift the ribs and torso up off the hips. Or you can do the tree pose with your back against the wall, for support and balance. You can also turn sideways and place a hand on the wall to maintain balance.

The benefits of Vrksasana include the following:

· It tones and strengthens legs muscles.
· It strengthens the ankles.
· It improves balance and coordination.
· It opens the hips.
· It lengthens the spine.
· It expands the chest for fuller breathing.

GARUDASANA

Garuda was an eagle deity in Indian mythology. In Garudasana, the eagle pose, the arms and legs are entwined.

Stand in Tadasana. Extend the arms out to the sides. Bring them to the centre and entwine the arms, crossing the left elbow over the inside of the right elbow. Turn the palms to face each other and join them. Lift the elbows to shoulder height and move the forearms away from the face to bring the wrists over the elbows. Bend the hips, knees and ankles as if you are sitting. Cross the left leg over the right thigh (SEE FIGURES 14-16 AND 14-17). Press the toes and balls of the left foot down on the floor. On an exhalation, lift the left foot off the ground and wrap the left shin and foot around the right calf as best you can. Gaze straight ahead. Observe your breath coming into and expanding the space between the shoulder blades. Hold the pose for several breaths and then return to Tadasana. Repeat on the other side.

FIGURE 14-16:
Garudasana:
front view

FIGURE 14-17:
Garudasana:
side view

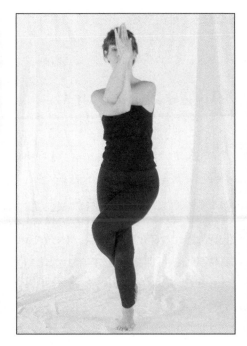
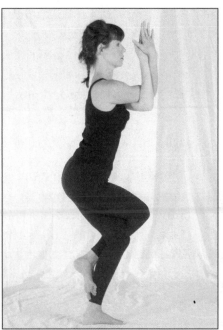

FIGURE 14-18:
Garudasana
variation

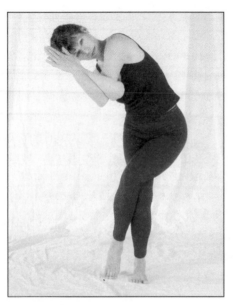

If your balance is precarious, keep the foot on the floor. If the hands do not join, hold onto a strap with each hand. You can also practise with your back lightly against the wall for support.

As a variation, once you're in the pose, exhale and bend to the right for several breaths (SEE FIGURE 14-18). Inhale and come back to the centre, and then exhale over to the left. Come back to the centre and then bend forwards from the hips. Inhale and come back up into the classic eagle pose to finish.

The benefits of Garudasana include the following:

· It improves circulation by squeezing and wringing out the arms and legs.
· It relieves shoulder stiffness.
· It strengthens the ankles.
· It helps reduce and prevent cramp in the calf muscles.

UTTHITA PADANGUSTHASANA I

Stand in Tadasana and press the feet down as you stretch up through the crown of the head. Spread the toes and the balls of the feet, and lift the inner and outer arches for support and rebounding of energy up the legs. Gaze softly ahead. Shift your weight onto your left foot, still maintaining Tadasana. Inhale and bend the right leg, lift the foot off the ground, and clasp the right big toe with the first and second fingers of the right hand (SEE FIGURE 14-19).

Re-establish the grounding of the left foot as you exhale and fully stretch the right leg in two directions, from the knee to the foot and from the knee to the hip. Try to maintain level hips. Release the bent-knee hip down and stabilize the standing leg. The right arm is also outstretched. Create a long spine and gaze ahead. Stay for a few breaths, then release and do the other side.

FIGURE 14-19:
Utthita
Padangusth-
asana I

FIGURE 14-20:
Modified
Utthita
Padangusth-
asana I

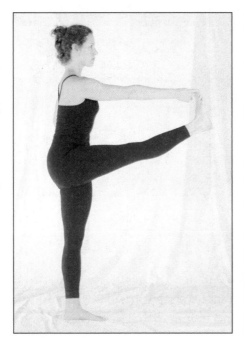
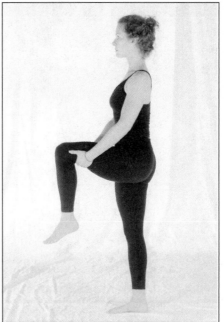

Instead of straightening the raised leg, you can also try keeping it bent and interlocking the fingers under the thigh, close to the knee (SEE FIGURE 14-20). Let the weight of the thigh come into the hands. Try to level your hips by releasing the bent knee hip down and strongly grounding the standing foot and stretching the standing leg.

Alternatively, try using a belt around the ball of the raised foot. Practise with the knee bent (SEE FIGURE 14-21, p 210) or extend the leg (SEE FIGURE 14-22, p 210).

FIGURE 14-21:
Utthita
Padangusth-
asana I
with belt

FIGURE 14-22:
Utthita
Padangusth-
asana I with
belt and
straight leg

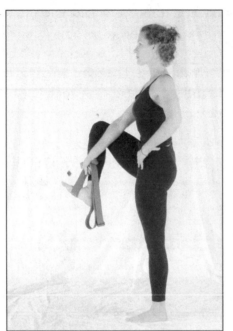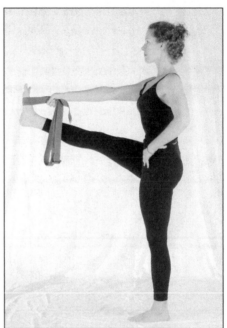

VASISTHASANA

Vasisthasana is the one-arm side balance. Come into downward-facing dog (Adho Mukha Svanasana). Place the right hand at the mid-line of the body (halfway to the left hand and in line with it) and the outside of the right foot on the floor. Lift the left hand off the floor and place it on the left hip as you place the left foot over the right foot, and turn the body to face sideways. Stack the ankles, hips and shoulders. Stretch actively through the feet and lengthen the front of the body from the pubis to the sternum. Keep the head in line with the spine. Extend the left arm up perpendicular to the floor and press down through the right hand, lengthening up through the right arm. Lift the right hip up, so it does not sag down (SEE FIGURE 14-23). Hold for several breaths and then come back into downward-facing dog, bend the knees and come down. Rest and repeat on the other side.

FIGURE 14-23:
Vasisthasana

FIGURE 14-24:
Vasisthasana
with upper leg
bent in front of
lower leg

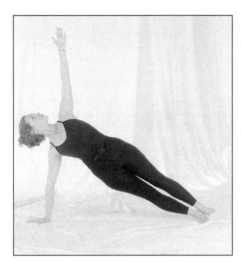

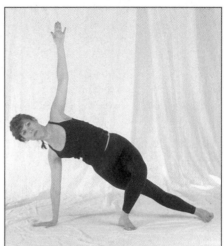

You can also try placing the feet against the wall for additional support and help with alignment. Alternatively, instead of bringing the upper leg on top of the lower leg, place the upper leg in front of the lower leg. Bend the leg and ground the foot onto the floor. Press through both feet (SEE FIGURE 14-24).

The benefits of Vasisthasana include the following:

· It develops coordination.
· It strengthens the wrists.
· It tones the lower spine.

CHAPTER 15
Backbends

Backbends open and lengthen the front body and loosen the shoulder and pelvic girdles. As the chest expands, more breath comes into the body. The groin stretches, which helps maintain length in the lower back for a healthy stretch of the lower back. The back muscles contract and strengthen to support the opening of the front body. Flexibility of the spine is enhanced. When done correctly, backbends heat up and open the body, and stimulate the kidneys and adrenal glands.

SPHINX POSE

Lie on your front with legs extended behind you. Prop yourself up on your forearms. Your forearms will be parallel to each other, with the elbows close to the waist and in line with the wrists and shoulders. Press the forearms and the palms down, and observe how this grounding action lifts the chest and elongates the sides of the body (SEE FIGURE 9-15, p 88). Maintaining this action, pull the elbows back on the floor without actually moving them. Feel the muscles of the upper back draw into the back and hug the shoulder blades. Enhance this by lifting the sternum forwards and up. Enjoy the openness and broadness of the chest. Hold for several breaths, then release down and rest.

The benefits of the sphinx pose include the following:

·   It strengthens the upper back muscles.
·   It opens the chest and stretches the muscles on the front body.
·   It teaches the basic back-bending action of coiling the spine.

If you are new to backbends you must start with simple poses, such as Salabhasana (locust), Viparita Dandasana (inverted staff pose) on a chair, Setu Bandhasana (bridge pose), and Bhujangasana (cobra). Once these are coming along well, more advanced backbends are suitable.

BHUJANGASANA

Bhujangasana is the cobra pose. Lie on your front with your forehead on the floor, your hands under your shoulders and your legs outstretched (together) behind you. Press the hands and the front of the feet down and lengthen the toes away from the body. Draw the elbows into the waist.

Inhale and look forwards. Stretch the chest, the area between the shoulder blades (upper back) and the ribs forward. The ribs and the stomach move away from the hips, and the hips stretch away from the legs. The pubic bone remains on the floor, and the lower back and coccyx lengthen away from the upper body. Space is created between the hips and the ribs, allowing the spine to lengthen into the body. The stomach receives a pleasant stretch.

Coil the spine into the body, like a wave that is moving in and up to arc before it spills over into the surf. Use your hands to press down into the floor to lengthen the arms up to support the coiling action of the spine (refer to FIGURE 13-27, p 185). The arms do not have to straighten, and they should not be used to create a push-up feeling (which will cause shortening of the lower back and compression).

Come up only as much as is comfortable for you. If there is lower-back discomfort, you have come up too far through the pushing-up action of the arms. The arms are there to open the chest more fully and to provide extra support. Hold the pose for a few breaths and then come down. Repeat several times, going up and coming down.

The coiling, wavelike action of the spine drawing in and up creates the backbend and the space between the vertebrae necessary for a safe backbend. The entire spine must be involved in stretching, or pain will be felt in the weaker parts of the back. The spine is like a cobra that slithers along the ground on its belly, with no limbs, and amazingly arcs up to strike its foe, with broad expansion and opening of its 'chest'.

As you coil the spine in and up, try letting the hands come off the floor (refer to FIGURE 13-28, p 186). Continue lengthening the upper back, chest and ribs forwards and up. Practising in this way will allow the upper back muscles to strengthen and draw in to support the spine and upper body. Without the use of the hands and arms, the lower back will remain spacious and long.

You may want to place a folded blanket under the lower stomach and hips (refer to FIGURE 13-29, p 186). Do the pose. The elevation of the lower abdomen and hips lessens the risk of lower back compression.

The cobra pose is not recommended for pregnant women. Those with lower-back pain should practice non-aggressively.

The benefits of Bhujangasana include the following:

· It stretches the front side of the body and its organs.
· It strengthens the spine and back muscles.
· It squeezes, tones and stimulates organs in the back body.

- It relieves backache.
- When done correctly and under the supervision of a qualified yoga professional, it can relieve sciatica and slipped disc.s

 People with cardiac disorders, high blood pressure and serious illnesses can do backbends. But these poses should only be done under the supervision of a qualified yoga professional, who will guide you through the poses and make sure you're doing them correctly.

URDHVA MUKHA SVANASANA

Urdhva Mukha Svanasana is upward-facing dog, the counterpose to downward-facing dog. It is a backbend, while downward-facing dog is a forward bend. Urdhva Mukha Svanasana has similar actions to cobra pose, the difference being that the legs come off the floor in upward-facing dog.

Lie down on your front. Extend the legs together behind you. Place your hands by your waist, fingers facing forwards. Stretch from the legs to the toes. Inhale and look forward. Extend your chest and upper back forwards and ribs forwards and up. Draw the ribs away from the stomach to create space for the spine to come in, lengthen and coil.

Press the hands and feet down to lift the legs slightly off the floor and to support the torso. Stretch into the toes as you continue coiling the spine forwards and up. Bring the upper arms back to draw the shoulder blades into the back (refer to FIGURE 13-30, p 188). Lift the kneecaps and firm the thighs. Gaze upward. Feel the stretch in the stomach. Stay in the pose for several breaths, then come down and release.

You can also tuck the toes under instead of coming up on the front of the feet (refer to FIGURE 13-31, p 188). This will stimulate muscle-hugging action in the legs.

When using the arms in the pose, bend the elbows out to the sides and press and lift the chest and upper back forwards. Then lengthen the arms. Do this several times. This enhances the expansion of the chest and the drawing in of the shoulder blades against the back.

If you have wrist problems, use support under the wrist to change the angle of flexion. Distribute the weight evenly throughout the hand. If you have lower-back pain, don't push aggressively into the pose. Create as much space as possible in the spine. Let the sacrum and coccyx lengthen down and away from the lower back. Often, the thighs lift too high off the ground, causing the lower back to pop up and shorten and compress. The thighs lift only in reaction to the pressing down of the feet (SEE FIGURE 13-31, p 188).

The benefits of Urdhva Mukha Svanasana include the following:

·   It's a wonderful stretch in the front body and its organs.
·   It's excellent for flexibility of the spine.
·   It strengthens the back muscles and spine.
·   It increases bone density.
·   It relieves backache such as sciatica and slipped discs.
·   It expands the chest and increases lung capacity.
·   It improves circulation in the pelvis.

Sometimes people feel nauseous from backbends, because of stretching the liver – this is normal. Holding the breath during backbends can cause headaches, underscoring the importance of continuous breathing throughout postures. After backbends, twists and gentle forward bends with a slightly rounded lower back are recommended to release the back and counterbalance the effects of backbending.

PURVOTTANASANA

Purvottanasana is the reverse plank pose. We will do preparation for the plank pose. Sit in Dandasana. Place the hands on the floor about 20cm away from the body, with the fingers facing forwards. Press the hands and the buttock bones and the back of the legs down. Bend the elbows and pull the arms back, letting the shoulders roll forward. Inhale and lift the chest and stretch the sides of the body up. Gaze straight ahead with soft eyes for several breaths (SEE FIGURE 15-1, p 218). Release and repeat.

FIGURE 15-1:
Preparation for
Purvott-
anasana

FIGURE 15-2:
On a bolster

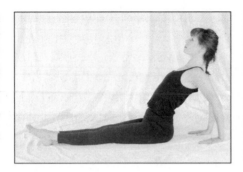
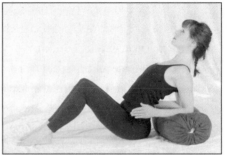

You can also try placing the forearms on a bolster or two vertically folded blankets (SEE FIGURE 15-2). Keep the knees bent with the feet flat on the floor. Press the upper arm bones down as you lift the sternum and top chest and stretch the ribs up. The pose can also be done with straight legs.

FIGURE 15-3:
Table pose

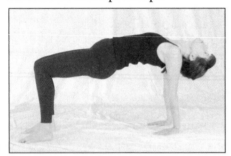

Try coming into preparation for Purvottansana, bending the knees and planting the feet on the floor. Inhale and lift the torso up so it is parallel to the floor. Stretch from the hips to the knees and from the hips up to the shoulders. Release the head and neck back if it is comfortable to do so (SEE FIGURE 15-3). This is called table pose.

The benefits of Purvottanasana include the following:

· It opens the chest fully and increases movement in the shoulder joints.
· It counterbalances forward bends.
· Table pose strengthens the wrists.

Repeat poses two to three times. Poses must be done gradually to build up strength and stamina and increase flexibility of the spine. There must be even extension on both sides of the body, otherwise compression is possible. The upper body extends away from the lower body. The sacrum and coccyx lengthen away from the lumbar spine.

SALABHASANA

Salabhasana is the locust pose. This is another prone backbend, which gradually arches the back.

Lie on the front with the legs together and extended. Stretch into the toes. Reach the arms out in front on the floor, with the palms facing each other. Stretch into the fingertips. Inhale, then exhale as you firm your abdominals. Keeping the abdominals firm, inhale and lift and extend the arms and legs. Keep breathing and lengthening into the fingers and toes (refer to FIGURE 13-32, p 189). Think of lengthening your front body without shortening your back body.

The head should be between the arms and at arm height. If the head is higher than the arms, the back of the neck will be shortened. After several breaths, exhale and release the pose. Rest on your front with your head to the side. Repeat two more times.

You can also start Salabhasana more gradually, to build up strength and stamina. First, inhale and lift the head (at arm height) and one arm. Exhale and release down. Then do the other arm (refer to FIGURE 13-33, p 189). Next, lift the right arm with the left leg, and then raise the left arm with the right leg (SEE FIGURE 13-34, p 190). The arms and legs can be raised separately. Lastly, raise the same arm with the same leg. Remember to lengthen and lift for extension, not for height or contraction of the lower back muscles.

Change the arm position. Bring the arms out to the side or clasped behind you, holding onto a belt. Stretch the chest up, and draw the shoulder blades into the back of the body.

The benefits of Salabhasana include the following:

·   It creates a long curve of the spine.
·   It strengthens the entire back side of the body.
·   It stimulates the spleen and the pancreas.

VIPARITA DANDASANA ON CHAIR

Viparita Dandasana is the inverted-staff pose. Place a chair, with the back of the chair facing the wall, 61–76cm (2ft–2ft 6in) away from the wall. Put a folded blanket horizontally across the front edge of the seat.

Sit down backward on the chair, bringing your legs one at a time through the space between the chair back and the chair seat. Sit in front of the blanket, with the hips close to the back of the chair and the buttock bones close to the back edge of the chair seat. Keep the legs bent with the feet flat on the floor. Hold onto the sides of the chair. Inhale and press down through the buttock bones and lengthen through the sides of the body.

Exhale, lie back on the chair, arch the back and slide the hips to the back of the seat. The buttocks are on the back edge of the chair seat and the wings of the shoulder blades are on the front edge of the chair.

Place the hands on the lower ribs and let the shoulders release down. Feel the chair seat supporting and creating space between the hips and the shoulders. Let the head relax down. Stay in this position for a few breaths to become accustomed to the pose.

Then, holding onto the sides of the chair, press the wings of the shoulder blades against the chair and lift the sternum up toward the ceiling. Press the hands against the sides of the chair back. Feel the chest open and the abdomen stretch (SEE FIGURE 15-4).

FIGURE 15-4:
With bent legs

FIGURE 15-5:
With extended legs

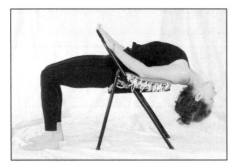
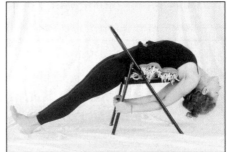

Last, bring the arms one at a time through the inside of the chair to hold onto the back legs of the chair. Extend the legs, pressing the balls and heels of the feet forwards (SEE FIGURE 15-5). The legs and feet remain active. Stretch from the front hips to the feet and from the hips, stretch the ribs away from the hips and roll the chest open.

Hold for several breaths. To come up, bring the arms back to the sides of the chair and bend the legs. Come up carefully, pressing the elbows into the chair seat while lifting the chest up. If your neck feels uncomfortable when starting to come up, use one of your hands on the back of the head to bring the chin to the chest as you come up. Put the forearms on the top of the chair back, and sit tall for several moments to counterbalance the posture.

FIGURE 15-6:
With bent legs
and head sup-
port

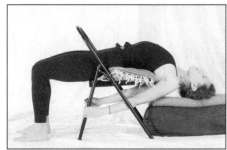

If you have lower-back discomfort, raise the feet onto a block or a low table. You can also change the height of the blankets if the back feels strained. For neck discomfort try supporting the head with bolsters or folded blankets (SEE FIGURE 15-6).

Do not practise this posture if you are experiencing a migraine headache or you have a tendency toward stress headaches. If you have insomnia, eye strain or dizziness, this posture isn't for you.

The benefits of Viparita Dandasana include the following:

- It increases flexibility of the spine.
- It calms and quietens the mind.
- It's soothing and relaxing to the brain.
- It increases lung capacity.
- It stimulates the adrenal, thyroid, pituitary and pineal glands.
- It massages and strengthens the heart.
- It reduces menstrual and menopausal symptoms.
- It relieves lower-back discomfort.
- It prevents varicose veins.

SETU BANDHASANA

Setu Bandhasana is a bridge pose. Lie on your back with the knees bent and feet flat on the floor, a little wider than hip-width apart. The arms are bent next to the waist, with the fingers stretching up to the ceiling. Palms face each other. Press the upper arms down for grounding to provide extension and length for the side ribs. Press the feet down as you lift the hips slightly off the floor (SEE FIGURE 15-7). Do not tuck your pelvis or press the pelvis up aggressively, as this will compress and jam the lower back. Imagine that the shape of the pelvis resembles a hammock.

FIGURE 15-7:
Preparation

FIGURE 15-8:
With inter-
locked
fingers

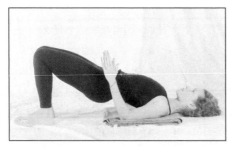 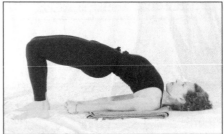

As you press the feet down, try to drag your heels back to your shoulders without actually moving them. This action will contract your hamstrings, lengthen your quadricep muscles and keep the strain out of your lower back. Support the lifting of the hips with the hamstrings and avoid overgripping of the buttocks. Breathe and hold the pose for several breaths. Release and come down with a neutral spine. Relax and then repeat the pose.

You can also try interlocking your fingers (SEE FIGURE 15-8),. rolling onto the outer edges of the upper arm. Or you can place a belt around the front of the ankles and hold onto each strap of the belt with your hands (SEE FIGURE 15-9). To support your back, you can also place a vertical block underneath the sacrum (SEE FIGURE 15-10).

Don't practise Setu Bandhasana during menstruation or pregnancy. If you suffer from lower-back pain, avoid this pose.

FIGURE 15-9:
With belt
around ankles

FIGURE 15-10:
With block
under sacrum

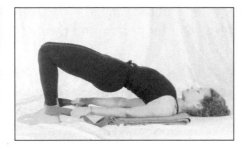 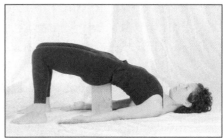

The benefits of Setu Bandhasana include the following:

· It's good preparation for shoulderstands and backbends.
· It increases flexibility of the spine.
· It stretches the front of the body, including the groin and thighs.
· It lengthens the back of the neck.
· It strengthens the back of the body.
· It stimulates thyroid and parathyroid glands.

SETU BANDHASANA SARVANGASANA

Setu Bandhasana Sarvangasana is another bridge pose. This is a restorative pose that provides similar benefits to the shoulderstand. In fact, it is good neck and upper body preparation for shoulderstand, as it stretches the neck and opens the chest, stretching the (often) tight upper chest muscles. Setu Bandhasana Sarvangasana can be substituted for shoulderstand during menstruation.

Place two bolsters vertically one behind the other (or use four to six blankets vertically folded) on the floor. Lie the whole body and legs on the bolsters, so the bottom edge of the shoulder blades are on the upper edge of the bolster. The tops of the shoulders roll down to the floor, doming and expanding the upper chest. The back of the head is on the floor. The arms can be diagonally by your sides, with the palms facing up, or they can be bent at the elbows, like a cactus (refer to FIGURE 14-8, p 197). The elbows will be in line with the shoulders.

Loop a belt firmly around the middle of the thighs, so they will not be able to roll apart. An extra belt can also be looped around the middle of the shins for extra support.

Close the eyes and relax. Remain in the pose from 5 to 15 minutes. To come out of the pose, bend the knees with feet flat on the floor and release the belt. Carefully move yourself in the direction of your head, until your back and buttocks are on the floor and your knees are bent (to rest your back). Then roll onto the right side and, using the hands, bring yourself up to a seated position.

You can also practise this pose by lowering the support under the torso for back comfort, raising the support to increase the intensity of the pose (if appropriate), pressing the feet into a wall to fully stretch the legs and open the groin, or placing a rolled blanket under the neck for support, to encourage and maintain the natural curve of the neck. This is beneficial for those whose cervical spine has flattened.

The benefits of Setu Bandhasana Sarvangasana include the following:

· It opens the chest and expands the lungs.
· It improves quality and volume of the breath.
· It stretches the front of the body.
· It lengthens the groin and stretches the psoas muscles.
· It calms and quietens the brain.
· It soothes the nervous system.
· It relieves backache.
· It increases blood circulation to arteries.
· It decreases insomnia and stress headaches.
· It improves digestion.
· It rests the legs.
· It prevents varicose veins.

CHAPTER 16

Practice Sequences

The practice sequences in this chapter are a guide to beginning a home practice. They are not a set of rigid sequences that must be done entirely or completely. Time how many breaths you take in one minute (most people take 16 to 18 breaths per minute) and use that as your base for the postures.

Fifteen-Minute Practice

The first sequence is a short 15-minute practice to get you started and for those days when you don't have much time to practise:

- Adho Mukha Svanasana (FIGURES 9-30, 9-31 and 9-32, p 99): do twice, for 30 seconds each time.
- Tadasana (FIGURE 10-1, p 104): do for one minute.
- Vrksasana (FIGURE 14-15, p 206): do twice each side, for 30 seconds each.
- Trikonasana (FIGURE 10-6, p 108): do twice each side, for 30 seconds each.
- Virabhadrasana I (FIGURE 10-10, p 112): do twice each side, for 30 seconds each.
- Viparita Karani (FIGURE 14-14, p 204): do for five minutes.
- Savasana (FIGURE 18-1, p 241): do for five minutes or more.

If a minute or 30 seconds seems too long to be in the pose, use your breath as the timer for how long you should stay in the pose. The breath should be steady. Start with five breaths for each pose, and, over time, work up to half a minute or one minute per posture.

Thirty-Minute Practice

The second sequence is a 30-minute practice focused on standing postures with some backbends, twists and an inversion:

- Adho Mukha Svanasana (FIGURES 9-30, 9-31 and 9-32, p 99): do three times, 30 seconds each time.
- Tadasana (FIGURE 10-1, p 104): do for one minute.
- Trikonasana (FIGURE 10-5, p 108): do twice each side, 30 seconds each time.
- Virabhadrasana I (FIGURE 10-10, p112): do twice each side, 30 seconds each time.
- Utthita Parsvakonasana (FIGURE 10-12, p 114): do twice each side, 30 seconds each time.

- Ardha Chandrasana (FIGURES 10-20–10-24, pp 116–21): do twice each side, 30 seconds each time.
- Salabhasana (FIGURE 13-32, p 189): do twice, 30 seconds each (the variations with single arm and leg raises can be done before, or instead of, the full pose, to build up strength and endurance).
- Bhujangasana (FIGURE 13-27, p 185): do three times, 30 seconds each time (do the full cobra depending upon your strength and flexibility).
- Supta Padangusthasana I (FIGURE 13-11, p 170): do twice each side, one minute each time.
- Supta Padangusthasana II (FIGURE 13-15, p 172): do twice each side, one minute each time.
- Jathara Parivartanasana (FIGURE 9-14, p 87): do twice each side, 30 seconds each side.
- Salamba Sarvangasana (FIGURE 14-4, p 194): do for three minutes.
- Savasana (FIGURE 18-1, p 241): do for five minutes or more.

Check your breath. If it is ragged and shallow or held, that means you're overexerting and need to back off, or you're thinking too much about being right. Try modifications of the poses and work up to the amount of time you can comfortably hold a pose. Be patient with yourself.

Forty-Five-Minute Practice

The third sequence is a more challenging combination of standing postures, backbends, inversions, twists and forward bends. As a warm-up, stand in Tadasana and interlock the fingers in front of you. Inhale and bring the arms overhead into Parvatasana. Stay for several breaths and then release and repeat, changing the interlock.

- Ardha Uttanasana (FIGURE 9-28, p 97): do for one minute.
- Adho Mukha Svanasana (FIGURES 9-30, 9-31 and 9-32, p 99): do three times, one minute each.

- Trikonasana (FIGURE 10-6, p 108): do for 30 seconds.
- Parivritta Trikonasana (FIGURE 10-7, p 110): do three times each side, 30 seconds each side.
- Virabhadrasana I (FIGURE 10-18, p 118): do twice each side, 30 seconds each.
- Parsvottanasana (FIGURE 10-26 or 10-27, pp 122–3): do three times each side, 30 seconds each time.
- Prasarita Padottanasana (FIGURES 10-31 and 10-32, p 125): do for one minute.
- Plank pose (FIGURE 13-25, p 181): do three times, 10 seconds each time.
- Chattaranga Dandasana (FIGURE 13-26, p 182): do three times, for a few seconds each (as long as you can hold the pose).
- Bhujangasana (FIGURE 13-27, p 185): do three times, 30 seconds each time.
- Urdhva Mukha Svanasana (FIGURE 13-30, p 188): do three times, 30 seconds each time.
- Chair Bharadvajasana (FIGURE 12-1, p 156): do twice each side, 30 seconds each time.
- Maricyasana III (FIGURE 12-2, p 158): do twice each side, 30 seconds each.
- Setu Bandhasana, supported (FIGURE 14-8, p 199): do for five minutes.
- Salamba Sarvangasana (FIGURE 14-4, p 194): do from one to five minutes, depending upon ease and comfort in pose.
- Janu Sirsasana (FIGURE 11-26, p 147): do once, one minute each side.
- Baddha Konasana (FIGURE 11-18, p 143): do once for two minutes.
- Upavistha Konasana (FIGURES 11-36 and 11-37, p 152): do once for one minute.
- Parsva Upavistha Konasana (FIGURE 11-39, p 153): do once for 30 seconds each side.
- Supta Baddha Konasana (FIGURE 13-1, p 163): do for five minutes.
- Savasana (FIGURE 18-1, p241): do for five minutes or more.

Once you have some familiarity with the poses, design your own sequences intuitively. Start with a pose and then see what your body feels like doing next. Honour your body and its innate wisdom. Let it teach and guide you. Experiment intelligently!

Restorative Practice

The last sequence is a restorative practice, meant to deeply rest and rejuvenate you. It is just as important as, if not more important than, an active practice. For more information about restorative poses, see the resources section and the book *Relax and Renew* by Judith Lasater.

· Adho Mukha Svanasana (FIGURES 9-30, 9-31 and 9-32, p 99): do with crown of head supported on block or blankets, for one minute.
· Prasarita Padottanasana (FIGURES 10-31 and 10-32, p 125): do with head support for one minute.
· Ardha Chandrasana (FIGURES 10-20–10-24, pp 112–21): do against a wall with lower hand on block, for one minute each side.
· Supta Padangusthasana II (FIGURES 13-15, p 172): do with foot on block against wall, two minutes each side.
· Supta Baddha Konasana (FIGURE 13-1, p 163): do for five minutes.
· Supta Virasana (FIGURE 13-2, p 164): do for five minutes.
· Balasana (FIGURE 9-20, p 91): place two or three vertically folded blankets between legs and under torso; turn the head to one side for half the pose and to the other side for the second half, for a total of five minutes.
· Viparita Karani (FIGURE 14-14, p 204): do for 5 to 10 minutes.
· Savasana (FIGURE 18-1, p 241): do for 5 to 10 minutes.

tips

Observe how your rate and quality of breathing change depending upon the type of pose you are practising. In standing poses, the breath tends to be shorter than in seated postures. The breath becomes even shorter when doing backbends and shorter still when performing twists. After doing a pose, stop and reflect on how you feel.

CHAPTER 17

The Classic Sun Salutation

A very popular vinyasa is the sun salutation, called *surya namaskar*, traditionally practised to greet the sun in the morning. There are many sun-salutation variations. This chapter covers the classic sun salutation, composed of 12 postures. The poses are forward bends and backbends, which create balance and equanimity. The forward and back bends are counterposes for each other.

PRACTISING THE SUN SALUTATION

Stand in Tadasana with your feet hip-width apart. Ground the active yoga feet and firm the thighs. Bring the hands into prayer position at the heart (SEE FIGURE 17-1). Gaze straight ahead.

FIGURE 17-1:
Tadasana with hands in namaste

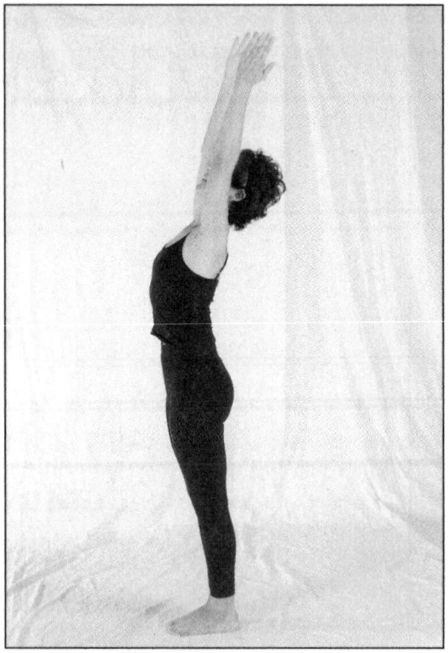

FIGURE 17-2:
Standing backbend

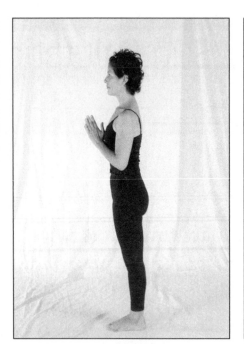

FIGURE 17-3:
Uttanasana

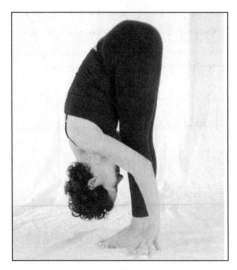

Inhale and extend the arms up over the head. Lift the heart, bring the shoulder blades onto the back and look up (SEE FIGURE 17-2). Keep the feet firmly planted down to move up.

Exhale and fold forward from the hips, extending the body and the arms forwards and down into Uttanasana (intense forward bend). Place the palms or fingertips on the floor by the feet (SEE FIGURE 17-3). Let the head drop.

Inhale, look forward and step the left leg back into a lunge (Ardha Mandalasana), with the toes tucked under. Bend the front leg at a 90° angle. Stretch into the back heel, lengthening the leg (SEE FIGURE 17-4).

FIGURE 17-4:
Ardha
Mandalasana

FIGURE 17-5:
Plank pose

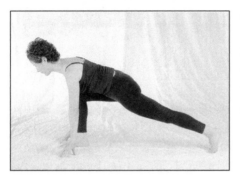 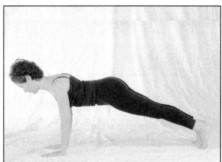

Step the right leg back next to the left leg, and come into plank pose (SEE FIGURE 17-5). Exhale and extend down into the heels, rebounding down into the feet and hands to move up, stretching the sternum forwards and keeping the legs and abdominals firm. Shoulders are over the wrists and hands are on the floor. Inhale.

Exhale and lower the knees, chest and chin to the floor. Arch the back, lift the buttocks and bend the elbows (SEE FIGURE 17-6).

FIGURE 17-6:
Knees, chest
and chin to the
floor

FIGURE 17-7:
Bhujangasana

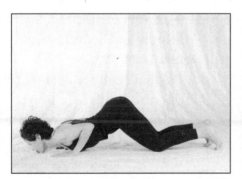 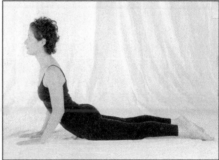

Inhale and glide the chin and chest through the arms, arch the back and press the hands down as you come up into Bhujangasana (cobra pose). Remember that it is the coiling of the spine and the lift of the body, rather than the pushing up with the arms, that brings you into cobra pose (SEE FIGURE 17-7).

FIGURE 17-8:
Adho Mukha
Svanasana

FIGURE 17-9:
Ardha
Mandalasana

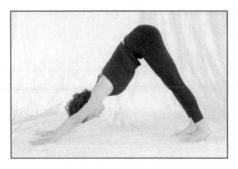
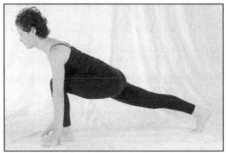

Tuck the toes under, lift the hips and buttocks and press the hands and feet down as you exhale and lengthen through the arms and legs to the buttock bones into Adho Mukha Svanasana (SEE FIGURE 17-8).

Inhale and lunge the left leg forwards, bending the knee over the heel as the right leg lengthens (SEE FIGURE 17-9). Hands are on either side of the left foot. Look forwards.

Bring the back leg forward to meet the front leg. Bend from the hips as you lengthen the spine. Exhale, and fold into Uttanasana, releasing the head and pressing the feet down, and lengthening and firming the legs. Palms are by the outside of the feet (refer to FIGURE 17-3, p 232).

FIGURE 17-10:
Standing back-
bend

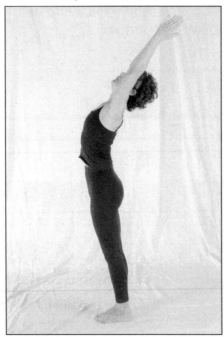

Inhale, extend the spine and the arms forwards and come up with a concave back and long legs. Raise the arms over the head, look up, lift the heart and arch the back (SEE FIGURE 17-10).

Exhale and return to Tadasana. Bring the hands into prayer position at the heart (refer to FIGURE 17-1, p 232). Repeat the sequence on the other side by lunging back with the right leg.

Initially repeat the classic sun salutation sequence on both sides, three or four times. This requires regular practice. As your stamina develops, increase the repetitions gradually, adding two extra rounds each week, and working up to 20 repetitions. Each complete round will take approximately two minutes.

You'll find that the flow and the rhythmic quality of your breath improve, and the breath becomes deeper and slower. Flexibility and strength increase, with greater range of motion in the spine and the major joints. The sequence provides aerobic benefit to the heart and lungs, tones and firms the body, and aids in weight loss.

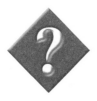

What is a vinyasa?

Vinyasa is made up of poses co-ordinated with breath in a flowing sequence. Vinyasa helps to heat up the body, similar to aerobic activity, and loosen the muscles and joints. It's a great way to warm up for a practice, or it can be an entire practice. Repetitions of vinyasa can build endurance, stamina, flexibility and strength.

MODIFICATIONS TO THE CLASSIC SUN SALUTATION

You can bend the knees slightly in Uttanasana (SEE FIGURE 17-11) and downward-facing dog (SEE FIGURE 17-12) if the hamstrings are tight or the lower back is weak. You can also bring the back knee to the floor when in the lunge position (SEE FIGURE 17-13, p 236), or let the knees stay on the floor in the plank position (SEE FIGURE 17-14, p 236).

FIGURE 17-11:
Uttanasana
with bent legs
and
long spine

FIGURE 17-12:
Adho Mukha
Svanasana with
bent legs

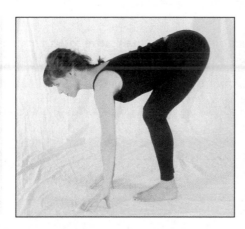
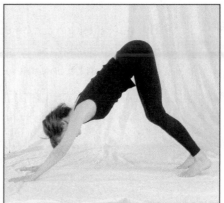

FIGURE 17-13:
Ardha Mandal-
asana with
bent back knee

FIGURE 17-14:
Plank with
bent knees

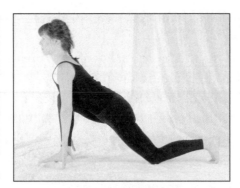
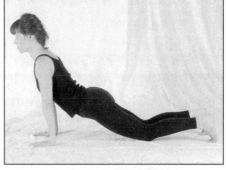

FIGURE 17-15:
Coming up
from
Uttanasana
with hands
on hips

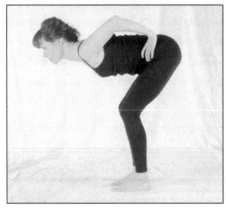

If it is difficult to bring the leg forwards from downward-facing dog into the lunge, use one of your hands to grasp the ankle and bring the foot under its knee. Another way is to bring the chin and chest forwards and up through the shoulders, while simultaneously swinging the back leg through into a lunge. This action creates space for the leg to come through.

Instead of extending the arms out in front of you when coming up from Uttanasana, you can also place the hands on the hips as you come up (SEE FIGURE 17-15), then extend the arms out to the sides and, finally, up over the head.

The sun salutation can be done slowly, with a meditative focus; it can be performed quickly, focusing on the flow of one pose to another; or the emphasis can be on the even, smooth flow of the breath. Several rounds of the salutation are very beneficial.

CHAPTER 18
Relaxation

The system of yoga provides many opportunities to develop relaxation techniques, which can help undo the effects of stress and tension. Deep relaxation is not a 'chilling out' activity, where you space out and let the mind wander or enter a sleep state. It is a state of alert consciousness that is deeply refreshing and energizing. The nervous system, respiratory system, circulatory system and digestive system receive the message to slow down, relax and regenerate.

The Benefits of Relaxation

We all lead busy, stressful lives. Our society and our educational system emphasize our abilities to think with our minds only and be cerebral. We are primarily valued for what we know, the level of education and expertise that we have, rather than for who we are. The ability to go within and become quiet and centred is not taught to us. Body education, in the form of physical education as taught in schools, misses the boat. Our minds are disconnected from our bodies. We don't know how to quieten and focus the mind. It is always active.

Daily relaxation is vital to optimal health, because it allows the mind and the body systems to rejuvenate and integrate the day's events. It is estimated that over a million Britons rely on tranquillizers to help them sleep. Insomnia is a growing problem that interferes with the body's natural mechanism for healing and rest.

Practising regularly is essential to experience the benefits of truly relaxing at a deep level. As you continue to practise deep relaxation, your awareness of how still the body and mind can become is heightened. In addition, there is an enhanced awareness of when tension arises. Relaxation begins to feel familiar and natural, while tension feels unnatural.

During deep relaxation, the body softens and the mind quietens, allowing distance and time off from our everyday worries and concerns. The relaxation response is connected to the parasympathetic nervous system, so when relaxation registers deep within the body and mind, the parasympathetic nervous system kicks in, producing sensations of tension release; slower, fuller breathing; slower heartbeat; and less firing of messages from the nervous system. The mind becomes calmer, with more space between noisy thoughts.

Often, students arise from deep relaxation feeling refreshed and rejuvenated, as if they had just been on a mini-break. It is important to realize that time can be very subjective and lose its linear perspective. Amazingly, a few minutes spent in deep relaxation can seem much longer, because of the immediate and lasting benefits experienced.

Many people report that practising deep relaxation improves the quality and amount of their sleep, reduces pain, relieves tension, helps manage stress, restores and maintains health, and engenders feelings of peace and acceptance. Deep relaxation and tension release also promote the suppleness of the body.

Through deep relaxation, you learn to switch from the 'doing' mode to the 'being' mode. This is not an easy process for most people. In our society, doing is highly valued, while 'doing nothing' is not accepted and may even be viewed as laziness or lack of ambition.

Most people think that they are relaxing when they are watching television, reading a book or taking a walk. However, this is not the deep relaxation we are talking about here. These are simply other activities of doing and thinking that allow you to shift gears slightly from your usual mode of doing. That is not to say that these activities aren't pleasurable or that they don't have intrinsic value. But these forms of relaxation are superficial, creating some quietening of the mind while the body may remain tense. There is not enough space between thoughts, and the breathing does not slow down enough to initiate the parasympathetic nervous system relaxation response. Of course, these activities can be enjoyable and entertaining and temporarily remove you from your ordinary reality.

The bottom line is that you need a balance between doing and being, otherwise you run the risk of burning out and becoming sick and disconnected from your true nature. When the sympathetic nervous system is constantly stimulated, your adrenal glands are overworked and depleted. Because they are perpetually on the run, many people eat unhealthy and non-nourishing fast foods, and do not listen to their body's requests to slow down and rest. Fatigue and sleep deprivation weaken the immune system, making you more susceptible to disease, as well as feeling tense and irritable. Your relationships can also suffer as a result.

The Basic Relaxation Pose

Savasana is the basic relaxation pose in yoga. In this posture, you learn the art of stillness of the mind and the body. It is typically done at the end of an asana practice in a reclining position.

The body is systematically relaxed, and this allows the mind to let go of the noisy thoughts that cloud perception and prevent total relaxation. During deep relaxation, you are practising and refining *pratyahara*, or withdrawal of the senses. It is this inward focus that is so essential to turning off external stimulation and enhancing relaxation. You are learning the art of 'being'.

Your eyes are closed and your breath is smooth and natural. Deep relaxation occurs while remaining conscious and aware of the entire process. The mind observes the relaxation process as a witness. Noisy thoughts come in and out of the consciousness and are watched dispassionately, as you would view a movie screen.

PERFORMING SAVASANA

The practice of Savasana also prepares the mind and body for *pranayama* (breathing techniques). The relaxation of the mind and body is important for a beneficial pranayama practice.

To practise Savasana, lie down with your legs extended and comfortable. Turn your palms up while externally rotating your upper arms. Have your arms rest slightly away from the sides of your body, allowing the armpit and sides of the body to feel open and soft, rather than hard and tense. (As an experiment, bring your arms right next to the body and feel the lack of softness and openness in these areas. Then bring the arms a little away from the body and feel the difference.) Use a folded blanket under the head and neck, if needed, so the forehead and chin are level with each other (SEE FIGURE 18-1). Balance the sides of the body, arms and legs, feeling equal weight on the shoulders, buttocks, arms and legs. Then release the effort. Inhale and exhale deeply, as if sighing, to release the body down to the floor.

Remain in this position throughout Savasana, with as little movement or disturbance as possible.

FIGURE 18-1:
Classic
Savasana

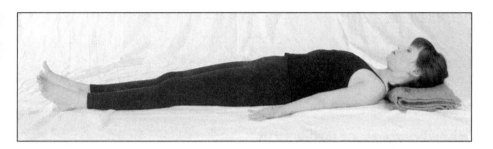

Begin scanning your body systematically, becoming aware of how you feel. Notice the quality of your breath becoming smooth, even and natural. Soften your eyes. Spread and soften your forehead skin and release your temples. Soften and spread your eyelid skin. From the bridge of your nose to the centre of your eyes, let the skin spread laterally to the hairline. Feel the heaviness of the front of your brain, full of noisy thoughts. Soften and release the front of the brain towards the back of the brain.

Soften your ears deep into the canal and relax the eardrums. Relax behind your cheekbones as you soften the cheek muscles. Melt the inside of your cheeks. Soften and spread your chin. Relax the throat muscles and soften the tongue. Allow your lips to touch and not touch.

Observe the heaviness of your body, arms and legs as your body begins to relax and let go. Soften the palms and fingers, the soles of the feet, and the toes. Relax the diaphragm and soften the front ribs. Soften your abdomen and release your lower back down to the floor.

Continue to release and soften. Relax your skin down to the deepest levels. Release the muscles down to their deepest levels. Feel the heaviness of your bones as they rest completely on the floor.

Observe yourself very slowly by systematically scanning the body. If your mind starts to drift, gently lead it back. As you continue to lie in Savasana, observe that the earlier heaviness of the body is no longer as noticeable. There may be a floating sensation, with the body feeling lighter. Remain in Savasana anywhere from 5 to 20 minutes.

Then deepen the next exhalation and lengthen the following inhalation, while keeping the brain quiet. Move your fingers and toes, and stretch your arms up over your head. Bend your knees and slowly roll onto your right side. Keep your eyes closed, press your hands down and use your arms to come up to a seated position. Let your head come up last, to maintain the state of deep relaxation. Slowly open your eyes and keep them soft and diffused. See if you can retain the inner focus and calm you have created.

Other Postures of Relaxation

Savasana can be practised following an asana practice, or any time you feel stressed out or fatigued. Conscious relaxation can also be practised in other supported postures, such as Supta Baddha Konasana (reclining bound-angle pose), Supta Virasana (reclining hero's pose), Viparita Karani (legs-up-the-wall pose), and supported Balasana (child's pose).

You can also practise Savasana with a bolster or a rolled blanket under your knees, or resting your calves on a chair seat. You may want to place an eye bag over the eyes, or stay warm by covering yourself with a blanket. Do not do Savasana if you're suffering from depression, mental illness or phobias, unless the chest is raised and supported.

The benefits of Savasana include the following:

- It soothes the nerves.
- It calms and quietens the mind.
- It diminishes migraines.
- It minimizes symptoms of chronic fatigue syndrome.
- It reduces insomnia.
- It aids in recovery from surgery or chronic illness.
- It removes fatigue.
- It integrates the effects of the asanas practised prior to Savasana.
- It prepares you for pranayama.
- It gives you an increased awareness regarding held areas of stress and tension.

Yoga Nidra

In Yoga Nidra, as we lie in Savasana, we systematically stretch and then squeeze the muscles before releasing and relaxing them. A chronically tightened muscle can be relaxed by stretching it and then making it even tighter. This exaggerated muscle tension sends a message to the muscle to let go and release at a deep level. Isolated muscle groups are consciously worked in this manner from the limbs up the body. We work from the toes to the feet to the legs and from the fingers to the palms to the arms.

Lie down in Savasana. Focus your attention on the right leg. Inhale and stretch the leg all the way from the hips to the toes. Then squeeze the right leg and observe all the muscles from the toes to the hips. Exhale and release the leg, allowing it to roll softly from side to side.
Let it relax. Repeat on the left leg.

Focus your attention on the right arm. Inhale and stretch the right arm away from the body, from the shoulders to the fingers. Make a fist with the right hand. Squeeze the right hand and arm and remain aware of all the muscles from the fingers to the shoulders. Repeat on the left arm.

Bring the awareness to the buttocks. Inhale and squeeze the buttocks. Feel the muscles on both buttocks. Exhale and relax the effort. Let the buttocks release and soften down to the floor.

Focus on the abdomen. Inhale and expand the stomach to capacity. Exhale and soften the stomach. Feel it recede towards the floor.

Travel up to the chest and lungs. Inhale and expand the chest and lungs. Exhale and let the chest and lungs relax. Feel the softening of the breath.

Move up to the shoulders. Inhale and draw the shoulders up to the ears. Exhale and release the shoulders away from the ears and down towards the floor. Let them relax.

Focus on the neck. Gently roll the neck from side to side and then back to the centre. Inhale and draw the chin toward the chest. Exhale and release the effort, allowing the head to come back to its normal position.

Travel to the face. Inhale and close and tighten the jaw. Exhale and soften the jaw.

Observe the lips. Inhale and squeeze the lips together. Exhale and relax the lips.

Move to the cheeks. Inhale and tighten the cheeks. Exhale and relax and melt the cheeks.

Become aware of the eyes. Inhale and squeeze the eyes shut. Exhale and release the eyes, allowing them to soften.

Focus on the area between the eyebrows and the forehead. Inhale and raise the eyebrows and furrow the brow. Exhale and smooth away the tension in the forehead and between the brows. Feel the whole physical body become heavy with relaxation as the muscles soften and melt down towards the floor.

CHAPTER 19
Pranayama

P ranayama is a powerful practice that controls and regulates the breath. It calms, strengthens and fine-tunes the respiratory and the nervous system, and increases lung capacity and elasticity. It has a calming and quietening effect upon the mind and the senses. According to yogis, when the breath comes under control, so too does the mind.

Why Practise Pranayama?

The purpose of doing pranayama is to distribute the *prana* (life force or energy) throughout the body. After asana practice, the body is open and ready to receive the prana. Potential blocks to the free flow of energy can be dissipated through asana and pranayama practice.

The energy channels in the body, called *nadis*, become purified by the change in blood chemistry caused by pranayama. Every cell in the body receives oxygen and nutrients and is nourished by these breathing practices.

Pranayama consists of inhalation *(puraka)*, exhalation *(recaka)* and retention *(kumbhaka)*. In pranayama, the duration of the breath is practised, with variable lengths of inhalation, retention and exhalation. The breath is very subtle and must be carefully developed and refined over time and regular practice.

Different styles of Hatha Yoga introduce pranayama at variable points in yoga practice. For example, Kundalini Yoga teaches powerful breathing techniques, along with asanas, from the beginning. Iyengar Yoga, on the other hand, carefully waits two years or more after a regular asana practice has been established, and the poses are steady and consciously performed. Neither system is right or wrong. The goal of Kundalini Yoga is to get the body's energy moving up the chakras. Their use of intense breathing practices, such as kapalabhati breathing, serve this purpose. Iyengar Yoga practitioners believe that the nervous system and the physical body must be made stable, strong and elastic, and its alignment must be correct before pranayama is introduced.

In this chapter, the major types of pranayama are introduced and explained. A supported lying-down position is usually the best position in which to begin, for the lungs are supported and open, and are less likely to be strained. As pranayama practice progresses, a seated position is beneficial. Then the spine is erect and the energy is free to flow up the spine.

Begin gradually, practising five minutes a day for two to three weeks, and slowly building to 20 to 25 minutes over several months. Practise up to three types of pranayama during a session. Daily practice is essential to build stamina, endurance and ease of breath. Then the lungs will be properly exercised and their capacity increased.

For the beginner pranayama is best practised prior to asana practice. If done soon after rising in the morning, the mind will be relatively quiet and free from distraction. Of course, it can also be practised at other times during the day in a quiet place. Pranayama can also be practised after asana, provided the asana practice is not strong and vigorous, as this disturbs the breath. A practice of quiet supported poses is conducive to breathing exercises. The advantage to practising pranayama after asana is that the body will be more open to receive the breath.

There should be at least 15 to 20 minutes of rest between asana and pranayama, or vice versa. After pranayama, it is appropriate to rest in Savasana or in some other restful position.

Pranayama should not be practised when tired or emotionally upset. The breath should never be forced or strained. If this occurs while practising pranayama, resume normal breathing and rest in Savasana.

Regular practice of Savasana (corpse pose) readies the body and mind for pranayama. Relaxation of the facial muscles, eyes, ears, tongue, upper palate and jaw is particularly important for breath work. The mind is freed from everyday concerns, allowing it to focus inwards.

Deep inhalations are not recommended for people with cardiac disorders or hypertension. The emphasis should be on the exhalation. Deep exhalations are not to be done by those who are depressed or who have low blood pressure. Instead, the emphasis will be on the inhalation.

Normal Breathing (Lying Down)

FIGURE 19-1:
Pranayama
lying down,
with support

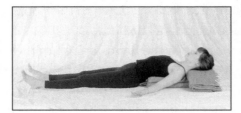

Lie on one or two blankets folded vertically. Place another folded blanket under the head and neck (SEE FIGURE 19-1). Close the eyes and soften them. Relax the facial muscles, jaw, tongue, upper palate and ears. Lie in Savasana for several minutes until you feel relaxed.

Observe your breath, noting the rise and fall of the chest and stomach upon inhalation and on exhalation. Note the natural rhythm of your breath, the length of your inhalation, exhalation and pauses in between. Slowly allow the breath to become smooth and even, so the length of the inhalation and exhalation is of similar length and volume.

Feel the mind start to slow down as the breath gradually deepens. Remain conscious and awake. Continue this exercise for five minutes. Then let the breath return to normal and rest in Savasana a few minutes.

You can also place a rolled blanket under the knees to ease the lower back, put an eye bag over the eyes to aid in *pratyahara* (withdrawal of the senses), or fold the blankets if you're pregnant.

The benefits of pranayama lying down include the following:

- It teaches observation of the breath.
- It relaxes the mind.

It is important to exhale completely before beginning a breathing cycle, and to end it on the inhalation. As a beginner, two to three pranayama breaths followed by three normal breaths and then two to three additional pranayama breaths is recommended. This prevents overexertion and fatigue.

Normal Breathing (Sitting)

Sit on two folded blankets in Sukhasana (refer to FIGURE 11-12, p 139). Cup the fingertips by the hips and lightly lift the buttocks and stretch the torso up to lengthen the spine and make space in the body for the breath to come in. Lower the buttocks back down to the floor while maintaining the length of the sides of the body.

Bend the elbows and place the back of the hands on top of the thighs, close to the hips. Press the buttock bones down as you lift and broaden the collarbones and stretch the sternum up. Draw the upper arms back slightly to bring the shoulder blades down and into the back. Bring the upper back in without jutting out the front ribs.

Inhale and lengthen through the back of the neck and the head. Exhale and bring the chin to the chest, by bending the neck forward at the seventh cervical vertebra (this is where the neck meets the shoulders). Close and soften the eyes. The chest remains lifted throughout the exercise.

Observe your breathing pattern, the length of the inhalation, exhalation and pauses in between. Be aware of the movement of the rib-cage, expanding with inhalation and contracting on exhalation. With each inhalation feel the rise and fall of the chest. The breath will fill the chest more than the abdomen. The abdomen does not inflate. Make sure the chest doesn't collapse when you exhale. Stay in this position for five minutes. Then lie down in Savasana.

You can also try this type of pranayama while sitting with your back against the wall for support. Or try sitting upright in a chair, without leaning against the chair back. Place the hands on top of the thighs.

Ujjayii Pranayama (Lying Down)

Ujjayii means 'victorious breath'. There are three ways you can practise Ujjayii Pranayama, depending on the depth on inhalation and exhalation.

Deep Inhalation and Normal Exhalation

Lie down on two blankets folded longways, with a folded blanket under the head and neck (refer to FIGURE 19-1, p 247). Begin with normal breathing and relaxation for several breaths. Exhale completely without strain. Inhale slowly, allowing the breath to deepen. Feel the ribs expanding laterally and the chest lifting as the inhalation fills the lungs. Exhale normally. Continue this breath for two more complete breaths. Inhale and then return to normal breathing for three complete breaths.

Exhale completely. Resume the cycle of deep inhalation and normal exhalation followed by three normal breaths. Repeat this pattern three times. Then lie in Savasana and relax.

You can gradually increase the number of cycles and decrease the normal breaths in between, according to the ease of breath you experience. Build up to 5 to 10 minutes duration.

Do not practice this type of pranayama if you suffer from a cardiac disorder or hypertension.

The benefits of this type of pranayama include the following:

- It increases the amount of oxygen taken into the body.
- It increases your energy level.
- It is beneficial for low blood pressure.
- It is good for asthma.
- It is helpful for depression.

Deep Exhalation and Normal Inhalation

Lie down on two blankets folded longways, with a folded blanket under the head and neck (refer to FIGURE 19-1, p 247). Begin with normal breathing and relaxation for several breaths. Exhale completely without strain. Inhale normally, filling the lungs and expanding the chest. Slowly exhale, and control the flow of breath as it leaves the body. The breath remains soft and smooth and without strain.

Continue this breath for two more complete breaths. Inhale and then return to normal breathing for three complete breaths. Exhale completely. Resume the cycle and repeat three more times, ending on the inhalation. Then rest in Savasana and breathe normally. Do not practise this type of pranayama if you are experiencing depression or low blood pressure.

The benefit of this type of pranayama include the following:

- It expels waste from the body.
- It soothes the nervous system.
- It quietens the mind.
- It is beneficial for cardiac disorders and hypertension.

Deep Inhalation and Deep Exhalation

Lie down on two blankets folded longways, with a folded blanket under the head and neck (refer to FIGURE 19-1, p 247). Begin with normal breathing and relaxation for several breaths. Exhale completely without strain.

Inhale slowly, filling the lungs and lifting and expanding the chest. Slowly exhale, and control the flow of breath as it leaves the body. The breath remains soft and smooth and without strain. Keep the inhalations and exhalations steady and even.

Continue this breath for two more complete breaths. Inhale and then return to normal breathing for three complete breaths. Exhale completely. Resume the cycle and repeat three more times, ending on the inhalation. Then rest in Savasana and breathe normally.

The benefits of this type of pranayama include the following:

· It fully oxygenates every cell in the body.
· It is very calming and relaxing.
· It is energizing.
· It soothes the nerves.

Ujjayii Pranayama (Sitting)

The following sections list three types of ujjayii pranayama in the seated position.

Deep Inhalation and Normal Exhalation

Sit for pranayama. Sit in on two folded blankets in Sukhasana (refer to FIGURE 11-12, p 139). Cup the fingertips by the hips and lightly lift the buttocks, stretching the torso up. Lower the buttocks back down to the floor while maintaining the lift and length of the sides of the body.

Bend the elbows and place the back of the hands on top of the thighs, close to the hips. Press the buttock bones down as you lift the spine up. Release the shoulder blades down as you firm them into the back. Bring the upper back in without jutting out the front ribs.

Inhale and lengthen the spine to the crown of the head. Exhale and bend the neck at the seventh cervical vertebra (this is where the neck meets the shoulders). Releasing the chin down, bring the chest to the chin. Close and soften the eyes. The chest remains lifted throughout the exercise.

Breathe normally for several breaths. Exhale completely and then inhale slowly, steadily and deeply. Lengthen the torso and fill the lungs. Keeping the chest lifted, exhale normally. Repeat this sequence twice more, and then breathe normally for three breaths.

Continue with two more cycles of deep inhalation and normal exhalation, ending on the inhalation. Then lift the head and breathe normally.

You can also practise this while sitting with your back to a wall for support. If you suffer from a cardiac disorder or hypertension, don't do this exercise.

The benefits of this type of pranayama include the following:

- It increases the amount of oxygen taken into the body.
- It increases your energy level.
- It is beneficial for low blood pressure.
- It is good for asthma.
- It is helpful for depression.

Normal Inhalation and Deep Exhalation

Sit for pranayama. Sit on two folded blankets in Sukhasana (refer to FIGURE 11-12, p 139). Cup the fingertips by the hips and lightly lift the buttocks, stretching the torso. Keeping the length created in the torso, lower the buttocks back down to the floor.

Bend the elbows and place the back of the hands on top of the thighs, close to the hips. Press the buttock bones down as you lift the spine. Release the shoulder blades down as you firm them into the back. Bring the upper back in without jutting out the front ribs.

Inhale and exhale, bending the neck at the seventh cervical vertebra (this is where the neck meets the shoulders). Release the chin down and bring the chest to the chin, keeping the chest lifted. Close and soften the eyes. The chest remains lifted throughout the exercise.

Breathe normally for several breaths. Exhale completely and then take a normal inhalation, followed by a deep, slow exhalation. Keep the spine lengthening . Repeat this pattern twice more and then return to normal breathing for three breaths.

Resume by exhaling completely, inhaling normally and exhaling slowly and fully. Do this entire cycle twice more. Then lift the head and breathe naturally.

You can also practise this while sitting against the wall for support. Don't practise if you're suffering depression or have low blood pressure.

The benefits of this type of pranayama include the following:

· It soothes the nervous system.
· It quietens the mind.
· It is beneficial for cardiac disorders and hypertension.
· It expels carbon dioxide waste from the body.

Deep Inhalation and Deep Exhalation

Sit for pranayama. Sit on two folded blankets in Sukhasana (refer to FIGURE 11-12, p 139). Cup the fingertips by the hips and lightly lift the buttocks off the floor and stretch the torso up. Lower the buttocks back down to the floor while maintaining the length of the sides of the body.

Bend the elbows and place the back of the hands on top of the thighs, close to the hips. Press the buttock bones down as you lift the spine up. Release the shoulder blades down as you firm them into the back. Bring the upper back in without jutting out the front ribs.

Inhale the breath, and lengthen up through the back of the neck and the head. Exhale and bend the neck at the seventh cervical vertebra (this is where the neck meets the shoulders). Release the chin down and bring the chest to the chin, keeping the chest lifted. Close and soften the eyes. The chest remains lifted throughout the exercise.

Breathe normally for several breaths. Exhale completely and then take a slow, deep inhalation, followed by a deep, full exhalation. Keep the chest lifted during the exhalation and the spine lengthening on the inhalation. Repeat this pattern twice more and then return to normal breathing for three breaths. Then start the lengthened inhalation and exhalation for two more rounds. Inhale and lift the head up. Relax. You can also try practising this while sitting against a wall for support and alignment.

The benefits of this type of pranayama include the following:

- The lungs are saturated with the breath.
- It soothes the nervous system.
- It reduces phlegm.

Kumbhaka

Kumbhaka is breath retention. In the following sections, there are several ways you can practise this.

Antara Kumbhaka

Antara Kumbhaka is retention of the breath after inhalation. Sit for pranayama. Close the eyes and take several normal breaths. Relax the facial muscles. Exhale completely. Inhale and draw the breath in from the pubis to the top of the collarbones. Expand the ribcage. At the top of the inhalation, pause and retain the breath, without tension. Feel the breath fill the lungs evenly. The lower abdomen draws slightly in and up. Keep the throat and the face soft. When ready, slowly exhale, releasing the breath. Take three normal breaths and then repeat the sequence twice more.

Don't practice Antara Kumbhaka if you have high blood pressure, hypertension or cardiac disorders.

The benefits of this type of pranayama include the following:

- It increases the amount of energy and oxygen received by the body.
- It increases vitality.
- It decreases fatigue.
- It's good for low blood pressure.

Viloma Breath

Viloma breathing is an interrupted breath, which is divided into segments, with pauses of breath retention between the segments. The breath is consciously spread to specific areas of the body. The breaths are divided into three parts in the following sections: from the pubis to the pelvic rim, from the pelvic rim to the diaphragm, and from the diaphragm to the collarbone.

Interrupted Inhalation and Long Exhalation (Lying Down)

Lie down on two blankets folded longways, with a folded blanket under the head and neck (refer to FIGURE 19-1, p 247). Begin with normal breathing and relaxation for several breaths. Close the eyes. Exhale completely. Inhale and fill the body from the pubis to the pelvic rim. Pause and retain the breath for several seconds. This will spread the breath throughout the pelvic area.

Inhale partially, filling the body from the pelvic rim to the diaphragm. Pause and retain the breath for a few seconds, allowing the breath to filter throughout the abdomen. Inhale from the diaphragm to the top of the collarbones. Open the chest and spread the ribs laterally. Pause for several seconds, expanding the breath throughout the chest cavity.

Exhale slowly and smoothly. Resume normal breathing for three breaths, then repeat the above sequence twice more. Gradually build up to six rounds of Viloma Breath. Relax in Savasana.

The benefits of this type of pranayama include the following:

- It increases lung capacity.
- It develops control of the breath.
- It decreases fatigue.
- It's beneficial for low blood pressure.

Interrupted Exhalation and Long Inhalation (Lying Down)

Lie down on two blankets folded longways, with a folded blanket under the head and neck (refer to FIGURE 19-1, p 247). Begin with normal breathing and relaxation for several breaths. Close the eyes. Exhale completely. Inhale and bring the breath in from the pubis to the collarbones. Keep the chest lifted throughout the exercise.

Exhale from the collarbones to the diaphragm and pause, retaining the breath for a few seconds. Try to keep the throat and the diaphragm soft. Exhale from the diaphragm to the pelvic rim. Pause and hold the breath for several seconds. Feel the abdomen spread with the exhalation.

Exhale completely, from the pelvic rim to the pubis. Pause. Inhale and take three normal breaths. Then resume, repeating the cycle twice more. With practice, gradually increase to six cycles. Afterwards, relax in Savasana.

The benefits of this type of pranayama include the following:

- It relaxes the mind.
- It makes the body feel light and full of ease.

Interrupted Inhalation and Exhalation (Lying Down)

This practice is suitable once interrupted inhalation and interrupted exhalation can be done with ease. Lie down on two blankets folded longways, with a folded blanket under the head and neck (refer to FIGURE 19-1, p 247). Begin with normal breathing and relaxation for several breaths. Close the eyes. Exhale completely. Inhale and fill the body from the pubis to the pelvic rim. Pause and retain the breath for several seconds. This will spread the breath throughout the pelvic area.

Inhale partially, filling the body from the pelvic rim to the diaphragm. Pause and retain the breath for a few seconds, allowing the breath to filter throughout the abdomen. Inhale from the diaphragm to the top of the collarbones. Open the chest and spread the ribs laterally. Pause for several seconds, expanding the breath throughout the chest cavity.

Exhale from the collarbones to the diaphragm and pause, retaining the breath for a few seconds. Try to keep the throat and the diaphragm soft. Exhale from the diaphragm to the pelvic rim. Pause and hold the breath for several seconds. Feel the abdomen flatten with the exhalation.

Exhale completely, from the pelvic rim to the pubis. Pause. Inhale and take three normal breaths. Then resume, repeating the cycle twice more. With practice, gradually increase to six cycles. Afterwards, relax in Savasana.

The benefits of this type of pranayama include the following:

- It develops endurance and stamina.
- It enhances relaxation, lightness and ease.

Interrupted Inhalation and Long Exhalation (Sitting)

Sit for pranayama on two folded blankets in Sukhasana (refer to FIGURE 11-12, p 139). Cup the fingertips by the hips and lightly lift the buttocks and stretch the torso up. Lower the buttocks back down to the floor while maintaining the length of the sides of the body.

Bend the elbows and place the back of the hands on top of the thighs, close to the hips. Press the buttock bones down as you lift the spine up. Release the shoulder blades down as you firm them into the back. Bring the upper back in without jutting out the front ribs.

Inhale and lengthen up through the back of the neck and the head. Exhale and bend the neck forward at the seventh cervical vertebra (this is where the neck meets the shoulders). Release the chin down by bringing the chest to the chin. Close and soften the eyes. The chest remains lifted throughout the exercise.

Begin with normal breathing and relaxation for several breaths. Close the eyes. Exhale completely. Inhale and fill the body from the pubis to the pelvic rim. Pause and retain the breath for several seconds. This will spread the breath throughout the pelvic area.

Inhale partially, filling the body from the pelvic rim to the diaphragm. Pause and retain the breath for a few seconds, allowing the breath to filter throughout the abdomen. Inhale from the diaphragm to the top of the collarbones. Open the chest and spread the ribs laterally. Pause for several seconds, expanding the breath throughout the chest cavity.

Exhale slowly and smoothly. Resume normal breathing for three breaths, then repeat the above sequence twice more. Gradually build up to six rounds of viloma breath. Relax in Savasana.

The benefits of this type of pranayama include the following:

- It increases lung capacity.
- It develops control of the breath.
- It decreases fatigue.
- It's beneficial for low blood pressure.

Interrupted Exhalation and Long Inhalation (Sitting)

Sit for pranayama on two folded blankets in Sukhasana (refer to FIGURE 11-12, p 139). Cup the fingertips by the hips and lightly lift the buttocks and stretch the torso up. Lower the buttocks back down to the floor while maintaining the length of the sides of the body.

Bend the elbows and place the back of the hands on top of the thighs, close to the hips. Press the buttock bones down as you lift the spine up. Release the shoulder blades down as you firm them into the back. Bring the upper back in without jutting out the front ribs.

Inhale and lengthen up through the back of the neck and the head. Exhale and bend the neck at the seventh cervical vertebra (this is where the neck meets the shoulders). Release the chin down by bringing the chest to the chin. Close and soften the eyes. The chest remains lifted throughout the exercise.

Begin with normal breathing and relaxation for several breaths. Close the eyes. Exhale completely. Inhale and bring the breath in from the pubis to the collarbones. Keep the chest lifted throughout the exercise. Exhale from the collarbones to the diaphragm and pause, retaining the breath for a few seconds. Try to keep the throat and the diaphragm soft. Exhale from the diaphragm to the pelvic rim. Pause and hold the breath for several seconds. Feel the abdomen flatten with the exhalation. Exhale completely, from the pelvic rim to the pubis. Pause. Inhale and take three normal breaths. Then resume, repeating the cycle twice more . With practice, gradually increase to six cycles. Afterwards, relax in Savasana.

The benefits of this type of pranayama include the following:

- It relaxes the mind.
- It makes the body feel light and full of ease.

Interrupted Inhalation and Exhalation (Sitting)

Sit for pranayama on two folded blankets in Sukhasana (refer to FIGURE 11-12, p 139). Cup the fingertips by the hips and lightly lift the buttocks and stretch the torso up. Lower the buttocks back down to the floor while maintaining the length of the sides of the body. Bend the elbows and place the back of the hands on top of the thighs, close to the hips. Press the buttock bones down as you lift the spine up. Release the shoulder blades down as you firm them into the back. Bring the upper back in without jutting out the front ribs.

Inhale, and lengthen up through the spine to the crown of the head. Exhale and bend the neck at the seventh cervical vertebra (this is where the neck meets the shoulders). Releasing the chin down to the chest, bring the chest to the chin. Close and soften the eyes. The chest remains lifted throughout the exercise.

Begin with normal breathing and relaxation for several breaths. Close the eyes. Exhale completely. Inhale and fill the body from the pubis to the pelvic rim. Pause and retain the breath for several seconds. This will spread the breath throughout the pelvic area.

Inhale partially, filling the body from the pelvic rim to the diaphragm. Pause and retain the breath for a few seconds, allowing the breath to filter throughout the abdomen. Inhale from the diaphragm to the top of the collarbones. Open the chest and spread the ribs laterally. Pause for several seconds, expanding. Pause and retain the breath for a few seconds, allowing the breath to filter throughout the abdomen.

Exhale from the collarbones to the diaphragm and pause, retaining the breath for a few seconds. Try to keep the throat and the diaphragm soft. Exhale from the diaphragm to the pelvic rim. Pause and hold the breath for several seconds. Feel the abdomen flatten with the exhalation. Exhale completely, from the pelvic rim to the pubis. Pause. Inhale and take three normal breaths. Then resume, repeating the cycle twice more. With practice, gradually increase to six cycles. Afterwards, relax in Savasana.

The benefits of this type of pranayama include the following:

·   It develops endurance and stamina.
·   It creates lightness and ease.

Nadi Shodhana

Nadi Shodhana is a form of pranayama in which the ring finger and the thumb are used alternately to partially close the nostrils on the inhalation and exhalation. The purpose is to cleanse and purify the *nadis* (energy channels). Alternate which nostril you begin the cycle with, so each side will be involved with inhalation and exhalation. The nadis will crisscross with the chakras, distributing prana to both hemispheres of the brain and every part of the body.

There are many variations in Nadi Shodhana, some of which include breath retention. The basic form of alternate nostril breathing is presented here.

Sit for pranayama. Raise and bend the right arm. Make a fist, with the palm facing the face. Place the thumb and ring finger with the little finger on the outside of the ridge of the nose (SEE FIGURE 19-2). Gently slide them down the nose until a slight indentation and the end of the cartilage is felt. Your finger will be above the nostrils. Practise applying light pressure on either side of the nose above the nostril, to partially close each nostril without moving the septum.

FIGURE 19-2:
Hand
position for
Nadi Shodhana

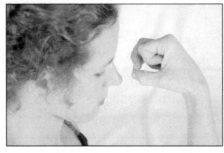

Begin with normal breathing and relax the facial muscles, ears, eyes and jaw. Exhale completely. Inhale through both nostrils. Close the right nostril with the right thumb as you slowly exhale through the left nostril. At the end of the exhalation, close the left nostril with the right ring finger and inhale smoothly and slowly through the right nostril. Repeat this cycle twice more. Then release the right arm to the lap and breathe normally for three complete breaths.

Exhale completely and inhale. On the next exhalation, close the left nostril with the right ring finger. Release the ring finger from the left nostril and close the right nostril with the right thumb as you inhale. Repeat this sequence twice more. Then begin the cycle with the left nostril closed while exhaling. Then lie down and relax in Savasana.

The benefits of this type of pranayama include the following:

· It results in a greater supply of oxygen to the blood.
· It purifies and calms the nerves.
· It quietens and clarifies the mind.

Kapalabhati Pranayama

Kapalabhati Pranayama is shining-face breathing. This form of pranayama is said to make the face luminous and glowing, and to cleanse the sinus cavities. Sit for pranayama and exhale completely. Inhale and then exhale forcefully as if you are blowing out candles with your nostril breath. Do this 10 to 20 times quickly, depending on your stamina and comfort. The forceful exhalation will draw the abdomen into the body and cause a spontaneous inhalation.

It is helpful, in the beginning, to place your palms lightly on the lower stomach. Then you can feel the lower abdominal area contract upon exhalation, moving away from the palms. This technique will help establish your natural rhythm for kapalabhati breathing.

Remember not to force or strain the breath. If you start to feel light-headed, stop and resume normal breathing. Work up gradually to as many repetitions as are comfortable for you to sustain.

Don't practise this form of breathing if you're pregnant or menstruating, or if you have eye or ear problems or high or low blood pressure.

The benefits of this type of pranayama include the following:

· It stimulates the liver, spleen and pancreas.
· It tones the abdominal muscles.
· It improves digestion.
· It drains the sinuses.
· It is exhilarating and a mood elevator.

Bhastrika Pranayama

Bhastrika Pranayama is bellows breathing. In this type of pranayama, the lungs and the abdominal muscles function like bellows, stoking the breath and heating and invigorating the body. Both the inhalation and the exhalation are forceful and vigorous. The sound coming from the nostrils sounds like bellows.

Sit for pranayama. Exhale any breath left in the lungs. Inhale quickly and sharply and then expel the breath quickly and strongly. This is one set of bhastrika breath. Repeat up to 10 times. Then rest in Savasana. Gradually build up the repetitions, never straining the breath.

Don't practise this type of breathing if you're pregnant or menstruating, or if you have high or low blood pressure.

The benefits of this type of pranayama include the following:

·   It stimulates the liver, spleen, and pancreas.
·   It tones the abdominal muscles.
·   It improves digestion.
·   It drains the sinuses.
·   It is exhilarating and a mood elevator.

Do you ever feel that your energy is drained by those around you? Practice bhastrika breathing. The rapid breathing, which consists of quick and intense inhalations and exhalations, will clear your energy field and help you feel revitalized and refreshed.

CHAPTER 20

Meditation

An important part of yoga is a practice called meditation. In this chapter, you'll find many methods for meditating, so you can find the method that works best for you.

What Is Meditation?

In the system of yoga, meditation can be viewed as the culmination of the limbs of *yama* (universal observances), *niyama* (personal attitudes), *asana* (physical postures), *pranayama* (breathing techniques), *pratyahara* (withdrawal of the senses) and *dharana* (concentration). Through the first four limbs, you develop:

- Moral and ethical conduct
- Physical health, resilience, flexibility, strength, stamina and endurance
- Vitality and energy through the distribution of prana

These limbs focus on the physical body, creating a strong, stable and clean body and a mind that is ready to begin meditation. They are the external path to yoga. The next two limbs – withdrawal of the senses and concentration – establish:

- The ability to turn inward and focus
- The ability to relax the mind and the body
- The ability to allow that concentration to spread and permeate the conscious intelligence throughout the entire body mind system

Then the mind becomes still enough to experience meditation. However, this does not mean that meditation will come easily. Like all other aspects of yoga, meditation requires commitment to a practice with patience. The other limbs have prepared you for meditation.

In yoga, meditation, or *dhyana,* is described as a state of pure, expanded consciousness. It is the seventh limb of yoga. The eighth and last limb is s*amadhi,* meaning 'freedom' or 'enlightenment'. *Dharana* (concentration), *dhyana* (meditation), and *samadhi* are the internal, subtle path of yoga called *samyama.*

Pratyahara (withdrawal of the senses) is the fifth limb of yoga that creates the bridge between the external and the internal world. Through pratyahara, you learn to disengage from the everyday world but remain aware and observant. This is commonly referred to as 'being in the world but not of it'. Without this detachment, it is not possible to meditate.

In meditation, you focus on an object for observation. As your concentration and involvement with the object deepen and your understanding of the object grows, the separation between yourself and the object seems to disappear. The unity of all things becomes apparent to you. This realization leads you further on the path toward *samadhi,* or self-realization.

The *Yoga Sutra* states that it is our misperception that we are separate from all things that causes our pain and suffering. Realizing that we are interconnected and interdependent, and that we are not alone, can lead us into a state of comfort and growth.

The Benefits of Meditation

Have you ever wondered why so many people try meditation when it seems so difficult to achieve? Perhaps a list of the many benefits of meditation will answer the question:

- Brain activity slows down (studies using EEGs, which measure brain activity, indicate that brain activity is much faster and erratic in a non-meditative state, but during meditation brain waves become slower and smoother).
- The mind is calmer.
- There is a slower rate of respiration; breathing deepens.
- Blood pressure is lower.
- The immune system is stronger.
- There are decreased levels of mental stress and body tension.
- There is an improved quality of sleep, and less sleep is required.

What does *om* mean?

Om is considered the sacred, universal, primordial sound. It is a symbol and sound of absolute reality. The *Mandukya Upanishad* says that *om* contains four parts: a, u, m, and the after sound (a nasal humming), which correlate to the four states of consciousness: consciousness, waking, dreaming and ultimate reality.

Different Ways to Meditate

There are a variety of ways to meditate. Different meditation techniques will work better for you than others. Just as some people are visual learners and others are auditory or tactile learners, different types of meditation appeal to different people, based upon their way of learning. Experiment with the different methods and choose the one you like best.

Soham means 'I am that'. It is a popular mantra that is co-ordinated with the breath. Soham is pronounced 'so-hum' and is thought to be the natural sound of the breath. It is very calming and grounding. During the inhalation, mentally say *so*, and when exhaling hear the sound *hum*. Each sound will be as long as the duration of each inhalation and exhalation.

Mantras

Mantras are sounds, words or phrases that are repeatedly recited in a conscious manner. The word *mantra* means 'to protect, guide or lead'. Mantras are used as tools for focusing during meditation. The practice of repeating the mantra, silently or audibly, is called *japas* (meaning 'muttering'). Mantras are meant to be repeated thousands of times, so you become deeply absorbed in the mantra's sound. After a while, the mantra seems to repeat itself. Then the mind becomes still and peaceful, uncluttered with noisy thoughts.

The mantra provides a backdrop for the true inner self to shine through. In some Hatha Yoga traditions, students receive a mantra from their teachers as a form of initiation. The mantra is kept secret and utilized only by the student. A mantra can be a Sanskrit word or phrase, or it can be any word that is inspiring, such as *love* or *joy*.

Chanting

Chanting also involves the use of sound. It is an extension of mantra. Chants frequently utilize prayers or affirmations as a way of entering into a meditative state. Chanting has a musical quality that includes rhythm and pitch, and has the potential to create an expanded state of consciousness. However, not everyone is comfortable chanting or reciting mantras.

Visualization and Guided Imagery

Visualization and guided imagery is another way to meditate, which is easy for beginners to learn. In times past, yogis meditated on their particular deity. Other suitable subjects for guided imagery and visualization are something in nature, such as a flower or the moon and the stars, or any scene, such as the beach at sunset or a golden meadow.

Gazing

Gazing is another meditative technique, where the practitioner focuses his open eyes upon an object for the length of the meditation. A common gazing object is a lit candle, although this is not recommended for people who suffer from epilepsy, and can really be any object. The gaze is soft and diffuse. It is not a hard, externally oriented stare, but a soft, internal gaze known as a *drishti*. The drishti is commonly used in several types of Hatha Yoga, such as Ashtanga Yoga, where each pose has a specific drishti to help direct and quieten the mind of the practitioner.

Focusing on the Breath

Focusing on the breath for meditation is another option. You can begin by counting breaths, as in pranayama practice. But a more effective way to use the breath, as a vehicle for meditation, is to impartially observe the breath. There are endless ways to do this. Some of these techniques are to:

- Observe the filling and emptying of the abdomen and chest during inhalation and exhalation.
- Observe the quality and texture of the breath. (Is it smooth or ragged, shallow or deep?)
- Focus on the breath as it enters the nostrils and leaves the nostrils.

Vipassana meditation is a Buddhist practice that observes the breath as its primary technique. It is popularly referred to as *insight* or *mindfulness* meditation. The word *vipassana* means 'to see clearly', 'to look deeply' or 'the place where the heart dwells'. Vipassana meditation believes that thought arises from the heart.

Observing Physical Sensations and Emotions

Observing a physical sensation or an emotion is yet another powerful meditative technique. Just as you would observe many different qualities of the breath – for example, its texture, substance, overall quality and depth – the same process would apply to watching physical sensations and emotions. The sensations and emotions would not be judged or altered in any way, shape or form. But your understanding and relationship to them could shift as a result of observation and meditation.

Walking Meditation

Walking can become a meditation as each step is taken consciously and carefully. You can:

- Observe how the heel reaches the ground before the ball of the foot.
- Be aware of the contact between the sole of your foot and the ground.
- Notice the texture and quality of the ground.
- Feel the shift in weight as you transfer from one leg to the other.
- Observe where your centre of gravity is with each step you take.
- Observe any thoughts that arise and let them flow through you without judging them.

Then bring your focus back to walking, step by step, foot by foot. Sit quietly after your walk, and observe your state of mind. Do you feel clearer, calmer?

Meditation Postures

There are two main postures for meditation: sitting and lying down.

Sitting

Sitting is the traditional posture for meditation. Sukhasana, or sitting upright in a chair, works best for beginners. Most important, as stated in the *Yoga Sutras,* a posture should be steady and comfortable. The spine remains long and erect, while the legs and buttocks are grounded.

It is a good idea to sit in Sukhasana (refer to FIGURE 11-12, p 139) on one or two folded blankets, to maintain the natural curve of the back and promote ease. You can also sit against the wall for support. If sitting on a chair, have your thighs supported by the chair and sit upright with the back of the seat supporting your back. Lengthen through the sides of the body, relax the arms and place the hands on top of the thighs. The palms can face up or down, depending upon which is more comfortable for you.

Bring the shoulder blades against your back to support and open your chest. Let the sternum lift and release the shoulders away from the ears. Lengthen up through the crown of the head, maintaining length in the neck. Relax the facial muscles and let the eyes close. The breath is smooth and natural.

Lying Down

Lying down for meditation has the advantage of being more relaxing for the body than a seated position. The disadvantage is that you might become so relaxed that you fall asleep instead of meditating! It can be a challenge to remain conscious and alert in a supine position.

You can lie flat on the floor, as in Savasana (refer to FIGURE 18-1, p 243), the basic relaxation posture. Or you can support the torso on one or two longways-folded blankets, with an additional folded blanket under the head and neck. The arms will be at your sides, with the palms facing up. The legs extend out of the pelvis and relax out to the sides. The eyes close and meditation begins.

CHAPTER 21

Special Applications of Yoga

The whole system of yoga can be utilized for therapeutic purposes. Yoga *cikitsa* (therapy) believes that we all have the inner resources to heal ourselves, but our attitudes, behaviour and lifestyle choices can adversely affect this natural healing mechanism and the desire for balance. The goal of yoga therapy is to help the individual feel better about him- or herself and to change attitudes and behaviour that contribute to the existing imbalance.

Menstrual Symptoms

Menstruation is a natural and healthy monthly cycle for women. However, it is also a time when many women feel tired and depleted. Menstrual symptoms such as nausea, headaches, abdominal heaviness and cramp, lower back pain and leg aches are common.

It is important to recognize and honour the need to slow down and practise a gentle, cooling and relaxing restorative yoga sequence. The abdomen should remain soft and inactive throughout your practice, so the natural menstrual process can continue unobstructed.

A yoga practice during menstruation emphasizes supported forward bends to control the flow of blood. Supported forward bends also calm and quieten the mind. In these poses, the back side of the body receives a beneficial stretch, which eases lower back discomfort, and the abdomen is rested and allowed to remain soft.

Supported, supine postures such as Supta Baddha Konasana (refer to FIGURE 13-1, p 163) and Supta Virasana (refer to FIGURE 13-2, p 164) help open the front body and the pelvic area and bathe these areas with fresh blood supply and nutrients. Inversions are not suitable during menstruation, as the flow will be reversed, which could cause complications, such as painful abdominal cramps and cessation of the normal menstrual flow before the natural process is complete. It is OK to resume inversions once the flow has stopped for eight hours. Unsupported backbends are too strenuous when menstruating. Twists, which wring out the abdomen, are unsuitable, since they squeeze the abdominal area and interfere with the natural discharge of menstrual fluid.

The following is a recommended sequence of poses for menstruation. The time you spend in each pose can be from one to three minutes, depending on your ease and comfort.

· Supta Baddha Konasana (FIGURE 13-1, p 163)
· Supta Virasana (FIGURE 13-2, p 164)
· Supta Padangusthasana II (FIGURE 13-15, p 172), with use of a belt and the outstretched foot supported on a block
· Baddha Konasana (FIGURE 11-18, p 143), with knees on blocks
· Upavistha Konasana (FIGURES 11-36 and 11-37—with bolster support, p 152)

- Supported Balasana (FIGURE 9-20, p 91), with long bolster or two to three vertically folded blankets under torso and head, turned to one side and then the other side for an equal period of time
- Sukhasana (FIGURE 11-12, p 139), with arms and forehead on chair seat
- Janu Sirsasana (FIGURE 11-26, p 147), with arms and forehead supported on a chair seat
- Paschimottanasana (FIGURE 11-32, p 150), with arms and forehead supported on chair seat
- Adho Mukha Svanasana (FIGURE 9-32, p 99), with block under crown of head for support and, if needed, a folded blanket to support the head
- Prasarita Padottanasana (FIGURE 10-31 and 10-32, p 125), with block under head for support (unless crown of head easily reaches the floor)
- Viparita Dandasana (FIGURE 15-6, p 221), with feet and half of shin supported by chair or bench and head on bolster or three vertically folded blankets
- Bharadvajasana on chair (FIGURE 12-1, p 156)
- Setu Bandhasana, supported (FIGURE 14-8, p 199)
- Savasana (FIGURE 18-1, p 243), with support under torso
- Ujjayii Pranayama Lying Down (see Chapter 19, p 249)
- Viloma Pranayama Lying Down (see Chapter 19, p 255)

tips

Remember that yoga therapy is not a substitute for traditional, allopathic medicine. The two can be used together wisely with good results. If you have any questions about yoga therapy, talk to a qualified yoga professional, and discuss your yoga with your doctor as well.

Pregnancy

Yoga helps prepare the body and the mind for labour and birth. It keeps the expectant mother healthy. Pregnancy is a great opportunity to let yourself relax and turn your attention inwards. Yoga can facilitate this process and help integrate the inevitable changes that come with new life. Your yoga practice can become the time that you devote to yourself.

Most of the asanas practiced normally can be done during pregnancy, with some modifications. Here are some of the benefits of doing yoga during pregnancy:

- The poses help keep the body strong yet supple as the pregnancy progresses.
- Yoga postures can strengthen the back muscles needed for support.
- Yoga postures can improve posture throughout pregnancy.
- Regular practice can minimize common symptoms of pregnancy, such as morning sickness, constipation, swelling, headache and toxemia.
- Pranayama practice will help decrease fatigue, stress and tension.
- When doing the modified poses correctly, there is plenty of room for the foetus to move about and continue growing freely.

Yoga postures and breathing practices teach you to centre and ground yourself. You learn to focus and concentrate. You learn the relaxation response. Breathing practices enhance your ability to control the breath and face pain with calmness and not fear. These are powerful skills for women during labour and childbirth.

Yoga practice should make you feel energetic and alive. If you feel fatigued, you may have worked too vigorously. During the first trimester, standing poses should be done without holding the pose for too long, as there may be feelings of unsteadiness or dizziness during this time. Avoid jumping the legs apart in standing postures. Standing poses after the first trimester should be done either with the back heel to the wall, against the wall or using a chair for support. It is not recommended to do asana practice from the 10th the 13th week of pregnancy, as this is a fragile time.

Standing postures help strengthen the legs, increase circulation and create energy, and may reduce leg cramp. Strong legs support and align the pelvis and spine correctly. As the leg and hip muscles stretch, their mobility and flexibility improve, and there is less stress on the lower back. Use a chair or wall for support in all standing poses.

While pregnant, it is important in pregnancy to keep the hamstrings stretched to avoid sciatica. It is also very important not to overstretch.

During pregnancy a hormone called *relaxin* is secreted, which loosens and softens the ligaments. If the ligaments become overstretched, joints such as the sacroiliac joint loosen, and instability and pain can result. Always practise with the intention of lengthening and extending the spine, to create space.

After the first trimester, reduce the amount of time spent in each asana, to prevent fatigue and overwork. For example, if you normally stay in a pose for 30 to 60 seconds, reduce the time to 15 or 20 seconds. Breathe continuously and smoothly. Keep the diaphragm soft.

When performing forward bends, do not compress the abdomen. Lengthen the spine and make it concave. This will maintain the length of the spine and make space for the foetus.

Supine poses can be done for the first three months. As the foetus grows, the additional weight can create pressure on the aorta and cut off blood supply to the baby. This is the major reason for stepping the blankets or lying in an inclined position.

During the second and third trimesters, supine poses can be done if the body is on an incline, by lying on folded blankets stacked like steps. Experienced yoga practitioners accustomed to doing inversions can continue during pregnancy. Usually, a woman is comfortable doing inversions until the seventh month, when the baby starts growing much bigger and the natural downward push of the baby is felt. Gentle backbends can also be done as long as you remain comfortable with them.

Deep relaxation at the end of an asana practice can be done lying on one side, with the top leg bent. It is nice to prop the head, the bent leg and its corresponding arm on pillows. Avoid poses that overstretch the abdomen. Bend forwards from the hips. In seated poses, a belt can be strapped around the feet, while the spine lengthens and the back remains in a concave position. This will help with lower back strain, especially as the baby grows bigger and heavier. Seated poses can also be done with the back against the wall.

Twisting poses can be done as long as the emphasis is on twisting from the upper back and shoulders. The abdomen should remain passive, as in Bharadvajasana (FIGURE 12-1, p 158).

Above all, listen to your body – if something does not feel good, do not do it.

The following poses are recommended for pregnancy (you do not have to do all the poses listed here every time you practise – pick and choose, depending upon your time and energy level):

- Utthita Trikonasana (FIGURE 10-5, p 108): extend both sides of the torso evenly. Let the hand rest on the shin or use a block behind the foot. Stay in the pose for 30 seconds early in the pregnancy. Then decrease the time to 15 seconds.
- Utthita Parsvakonasana (FIGURE 10-12, p 114): follow the suggestions for Utthita Trikonasana.
- Virabhadrasana I (FIGURE 10-10, p 112): do not bend the front leg so deeply. Spend less time in the pose. Extend the spine and look straight ahead. Stay for 10 to 15 seconds per side.
- Virabhadrasana II (FIGURE 10-18, p 118): same as for Virabhadrasana I.
- Ardha Chandrasana (FIGURE 10-23, p 121): place the palm on a block or use a chair or wall for support. Keep the pelvis broad. Stay for 10 to 15 seconds on each side. This pose helps with morning sickness.
- Parsvottanasana (FIGURE 10-26, p 122): keep the torso parallel to the floor. Extend from the pubis to the sternum. Place the hands on a chair seat or the top of the chair back. Stay for 10 to 15 seconds on each side.
- Prasarita Padottanasana (FIGURE 10-31, p 125): extend the spine towards the head and press the thighs back to make the spine concave. Stretch the arms. Place the hands on blocks or a chair seat. Hold the pose for 15 to 20 seconds. This pose helps with morning sickness.
- Janu Sirsasana (FIGURE 11-26, p 147): use a belt around the outstretched foot. Hold onto the belt with both hands, pressing the top of the straight leg down, lift up through the spine, bringing the back body to the front body to make it concave. Look up. Remain in the pose 10 to 15 seconds on each side. This pose strengthens the spine and the back and waist muscles, and is good for supporting the foetus.
- Baddha Konasana (FIGURE 11-18, p 143): the back can rest on the wall, with the arms by the sides and palms or fingertips on the floor.

- Supta Baddha Konasana (FIGURE 13-1, p 163): fold the blankets and use blocks for support under the thighs. Stay in the pose for as long as you are comfortable. This is a great resting pose that opens the pelvis.
- Upavistha Konasana (FIGURES 11-36 and 11-37, p 152): sit on folded blankets with your back to the wall for as long as is comfortable. Bend the knees and bring the legs together to come out of the pose without straining the groin.

The following poses facilitate an easier delivery. They also strengthen the spine:

- Virasana (FIGURE 11-9, p 137): sit with a folded blanket or two under the buttocks, so the uterus will not press down. Stay in the pose as long as it is comfortable. Virasana helps decrease swelling and prevents varicose veins, which are common in pregnancy.
- Supta Virasana (FIGURE 13-2, p 164): elevate the torso on stacked and folded blankets, so the head and torso are higher than the thighs. Arms can be overhead or by the torso. Stay as long as it is comfortable. This posture relieves morning sickness, constipation and wind, and decreases swelling.
- Parvatasana (FIGURE 11-8, p 136): sit on a folded blanket. This asana helps the kidneys function optimally.
- Sirsasana (FIGURE 14-11 and 14-13, pp 202–3): this pose can be done *only if* you regularly practise it. It can be done with or without support. Stay in the pose from 3 to 5 minutes. Do not practise if the chest feels heavy or the heart beats faster than normal.
- Sarvangasana (FIGURE 14-15, p 206) same as for Sirsasana. Sarvangasana calms the mind, soothes the nerves and is helpful in cases of toxemia.
- Halasana (FIGURE 14-2, p 194): can be done by an experienced practitioner. After three months the feet must be elevated on a chair to keep the abdomen from being compressed. Can be done up until the seventh month. Keep the legs wide enough apart to give the abdomen adequate space. Do not do the pose if pressure is felt in the chest or if the womb is compressed.

- Bharadvajasana on a Chair (FIGURE 12-1, p 156): can be done up until the seventh month. This asana strengthens the lower spine and the waist muscles.

During pregnancy, pranayama and savasana are invaluable for health and vitality. They calm the mind, soothe the nerves and strengthen the body. Pranayama can be done either lying down with stacked, folded blankets, or seated with wall support. Ujjayii Pranayama lying down and Viloma Pranayama lying down and seated are wonderful during pregnancy and help reduce labour spasms and strains.

For additional information about yoga and pregnancy books, refer to the bibliography at the end of this book, or try *www.amazon.co.uk*. Many of the ideas and postures in this section were inspired by *Yoga: A Gem for Women* by Geeta Iyengar, *Preparing for Birth with Yoga* by Janet Balaskas and *Yoga for Pregnancy* by Sandra Jordan.

Perimenopause and Menopause Sequence

The cessation of the menstrual cycle usually occurs between the ages of 45 and 55 years of age. Menopause can happen gradually or abruptly. Many women experience perimenopausal symptoms prior to actual menopause. During this time, levels of progesterone and oestrogen become uneven. The symptoms include:

- Disrupted sleep patterns
- Lack of energy
- Mental fuzziness and trouble concentrating
- Weight gain
- Osteoporosis
- Hot flushes
- Night sweats
- Mood swings
- Heart palpitations

- Changes in menstruation, such as heavier bleeding, spotting and skipping of periods
- Racy, manic tendencies prior to menstruation

Yoga can help alleviate some of these symptoms and ease the transition into menopause. Postures keep the reproductive glands balanced and nourished. The following sequence is appropriate for perimenopausal and menopausal women. Poses can be done for up to 5 minutes each, according to your capacity:

- Upavistha Konasana (FIGURES 11-36 and 11-37, p 152)
- Baddha Konasana (FIGURE 11-18, p 143)
- Vajrasana (FIGURE 11-5, p 135), with toes tucked under and rolled mat between calves and back of thighs
- Supta Baddha Konasana (FIGURE 13-1, p 163), supported
- Virasana (FIGURE 11-9, p 137)
- Supta Virasana (FIGURE 13-2, p 164)
- Supta Vrksasana (FIGURE 9-1, p 80), with feet against wall
- Supta Padangusthasana I (FIGURE 13-11, p 170), with belt and foot against wall
- Supta Padangusthasana II (FIGURE 13-15, p 172), with belt and foot against wall
- Prasarita Padottanasana (FIGURE 10-31, p 125)
- Adho Mukha Svanasana (FIGURE 9-32, p 99), with head supported
- Uttanasana (FIGURE 10-34 and 10-35, p 127), with support under head, arms folded, holding onto elbows with hands
- Utthita Trikonasana (FIGURE 10-5, p 108), with back outer foot against wall
- Parsvottanasana (FIGURE 10-25, p 123), with back outer foot against wall
- Virabhadrasana I (FIGURE 10-10, p 112), with back outer foot against wall
- Ardha Chandrasana (FIGURE 10-23, p 121), with back foot on wall, hand on vertical block, and standing foot by centreline of mat, back foot to wall
- Supported Balasana (FIGURE 9-20, p 91)
- Janu Sirsasana (FIGURE 11-26, p 147), with head and arms resting on chair seat
- Paschimottanasana (FIGURE 11-32, p 150), with head resting on several blankets
- Sirsasana (FIGURE 14-10, p 201 or 14-13, p 203)

- Viparita Dandasana (FIGURE 15-4 and 15-5, p 220)
- Sarvangasana (FIGURE 14-1–14-5, pp 192–5), with chair and three blankets
- Halasana (FIGURE 14-6, p 196), with legs on chair
- Setu Bandhasana (FIGURE 14-8, p 199), supported with two bolsters and a belt around the thighs
- Viparita Karani (FIGURE 14-14, p 204), with bolster
- Savasana (FIGURE 18-1, p 241), with support
- Ujjayii Pranayama (see Chapter 19, p 249)
- Viloma Pranayama (see Chapter 19, p 255)

Partner Yoga is a playful way to enjoy practising yoga. Most partner poses involve mirroring the pose to each other (for example, doing tree pose with the straight-legged side of the body in contact with your partner's side). Partner Yoga requires communication and feedback between partners and is, therefore, an opportunity to develop your clarity of thought and speech.

Yoga for Men

Yoga is as beneficial for men as it is for women. It can help balance an exercise programme that includes weight training and aerobic activity. The combination of developing flexibility, strength, stamina and the ability to focus and relax and to decrease stress, is unbeatable. Many men claim that their yoga practice helps their performance and concentration at work, as well as in sports. And after several months of practice, many experience weight loss and redistribution of fat. Yoga also develops the body-mind connection, vital to overall health and intimacy with oneself and others.

As men age, they are also subject to a variety of common problems, such as insomnia, impotence and prostate conditions. Men may even undergo a male menopause, with changes and disruptions in hormonal levels, just like women. It's just not as noticeable as women's changes.

Men have more muscle mass than women, and therefore tend to have greater tightness and restriction in the hips, shoulders, hamstrings and groin. Many sports, such as golf and tennis, create imbalances as a result of their one-sided natures. Yoga helps correct these asymmetries. The following is a sequence designed to minimize these conditions and balance the health of the reproductive organs:

- Ardha Chandrasana (FIGURE 10-24, p 121), with a block
- Trikonasana (FIGURE 10-4, p 108)
- Utthita Parsvakonasana (FIGURE 10-12, p 114)
- Virabhadrasana II (FIGURE 10-18, p 118)
- Baddha Konasana (FIGURE 11-18, p 143), with blocks under knees and hand behind buttocks, using wall for back support if desired
- Upavistha Konasana (FIGURES 11-36 and 11-37, p 152), with hands by hips, using wall for back support if desired
- Navasana (FIGURE 11-22, p 145)
- Janu Sirsasana (FIGURE 11-26, p 147), with concave back, looking up
- Viparita Dandasana (FIGURE 15-4, p 220), on chair, with block under feet against wall
- Supta Virasana (FIGURE 13-2, p 164), with support
- Supta Baddha Konasana (FIGURE 13-1, p 163), with support
- Bharadvajasana (FIGURE 12-1, p 156)
- Supta Padangusthasana II (FIGURE 13-15, p 172), with block under foot
- Sirsasana (FIGURE 14-11 or 14-12, p 202)
- Sarvangasana (FIGURE 14-1, p 192)
- Setu Bandhasana (FIGURE 14-8, p 199), with support
- Halasana (FIGURE 14-2, p 194), with a chair
- Viparita Karani (FIGURE 14-14, p 204)
- Savasana (FIGURE 18-1, p 241), with support under calves
- Ujjayii Pranayama Lying Down (see Chapter 19, p 249)
- Viloma Pranayama Lying Down (see Chapter 19, p 255)

Scoliosis

Scoliosis is a condition in which there is curvature of the spine. It can be functional, a curvature that is not inherent in the structure of the spine, but is the result of other factors, such as imbalances elsewhere in the body, for example in the pelvis. With functional scoliosis the curvature may disappear when one bends forward.

True scoliosis is a curvature that is part of the structure of the spine. With true scoliosis it is possible to observe that one side of the back rib cage protrudes more than the other side, one shoulder may be higher than the other or one side of the pelvis is higher. There are parts of the spine that are concave and convex, creating misalignment, collapse and overstretching simultaneously.

For someone with scoliosis, it is crucial to lengthen and strengthen the supporting muscles of the spine for relief of pain, tightness and compression. Many yoga poses elongate the spine and the *paraspinal muscles* (the long muscles down the spine), while other (supporting) back muscles are strengthened. This helps prevent further lateral curvature and rotation.

Standing postures strengthen the legs and build a solid foundation from which the pelvis balances and the spine can then stretch freely out of the pelvis. The legs must carry the weight of the body, not the spine.

Flexibility and mobility in the hips and legs are also necessary for a range of motion and good posture. Very often the upper back muscles are very tight, especially the *trapezius muscle,* the big muscle from the neck to the bottom of the shoulder blade.

Learning to breathe into the tight side of the body to increase lung capacity is essential. The compression on the concave side tightens the intercostal muscles between the ribs, and therefore leads to diminished breathing capacity. Suggested yoga poses for scoliosis include the following:

- Ardha Uttanasana (FIGURE 9-28, p 97)
- Squatting while holding onto a table or counter
- Cat pose – alternately rounding and arching the back with the breath while on all fours (FIGURES 9-18 and 9-19, pp 90–1)
- Balasana (FIGURE 9-20, p 91)
- Ardha Mandalasana (FIGURE 9-27, p 96)
- Raja Kapotasana (FIGURES 13-22 and 13-23, p 79)
- Supta Padangusthasana I (FIGURES 13-11 and 13-12, p 170)
- Stomach turning pose with bottom leg straight

- Basic relaxation pose with towel or hand towel under concave side of back

Sciatica

The sciatic nerve is the longest and largest nerve, beginning in the lower back and continuing through each thigh, calf and foot. When the sciatic nerve becomes irritated and inflamed, radiating pain can be felt in the lower back, thighs, calves and feet. Sensations of sharp or burning pain as well as pins and needles, numbness, tingling, prickliness and tenderness may be experienced. Sometimes, the pain is felt in only one leg; in other cases the pain radiates down both legs.

Frequently, the cause of sciatica is a herniated disc in the lower back that compresses one of the nerve roots of the sciatic nerve. Another cause of sciatic pain is a tight piriformis muscle impinging on the sciatic nerve and causing irritation of the nerve. The piriformis muscle encompasses the space between the sacrum and the upper end of the thighbone, crossing over the sciatic nerve. This muscle works on the leg at the hip joint, and rotates the thighs externally so the toes point out away from the mid-line of the body. People who stand with their toes turned out, and cyclists and runners with continually contracted, overworked and understretched piriformis muscles are prime candidates for sciatica. Unbalanced posture in daily life, where weight is unevenly distributed on both feet when standing or walking, or unevenly on both buttock bones while seated, will in time cause imbalances in the pelvis area and can lead to nerve-related problems such as sciatica.

The following are postures recommended for relief of sciatic pain. They are based upon an Iyengar Yoga therapeutic sequence:

- *Dandasana* (FIGURE 11-1, p 128), with weights. Sit with a long, upright spine, with the legs straight out in front of you. Put a blanket or pillow on the affected thigh and on top of it a weight of 9–11kg (20–25lb). Stay in the posture for several minutes.
- *Utthita Hasta Padangusthasana II*. Stand in Tadasana facing a counter. Transfer the weight onto the left leg and foot, and line up the outer hip over the ankle. Raise the right leg and place it on the counter. The back of the right leg, including the hip, will be on the counter. If

the bottom of the hip does not reach the counter, place a folded blanket or towel under it for support. Place a weight of 4.5 to 6.7kg (10 to 15lb) on top of the right thigh. This will calm the irritated sciatic nerve so it elongates and relaxes. Draw the right leg back into the hip socket as you extend into the foot. Extend up evenly on both sides of the body and try to keep the hips level with one another. Hold the pose for one minute. Release and repeat on the other side.

- *Standing Marichyasana.* Place a stool next to a wall. Stand behind the stool with the left side of the body next to the wall. Put the left foot on the stool with the knee bent to slightly higher than 90°. The left foot should be in line with or slightly higher than the left hip. A wooden block (or a book) can be placed under the right heel to elevate it. The right foot is facing the stool, with the toes pointing straight ahead. Inhale and lengthen the spine. Exhale and turn the body toward the wall, placing the fingertips of each hand on the wall at shoulder height, but wider apart than the shoulders. As you continue inhaling and lengthening, exhaling and revolving toward the wall, see if you can have your shoulders and chest parallel to the wall. After several breaths in this position, slowly unwind and release. It is important to move slowly and with awareness. Moving quickly often leads to injury. Then repeat on the other side. Standing Marichyasana should be done twice on both sides for short periods of time (not held for too long).

- *Supta Padangusthasana I* (FIGURE 13-11, p 170). Lie down and extend the legs on the floor. Stretching into the feet, lengthen into the crown of the head. Bend the right leg and extend it up to perpendicular, with the sole of the foot facing the ceiling. Hold onto the foot with a belt around the arch and the hands holding each side of the belt. Press the back of the left leg down, unless straightening the leg would cause pain. Instead, bend the bottom leg. Feel the thigh muscles hug the bone. Lengthen the inner and outer heels away from the ankles, spread the toes and lift the inner and outer arches. Draw this action up the legs. Lengthen your outer right hip away from the right armpit. Feel the action drawing up the legs. Elongate the sides of the body from the hips to the armpits. Lengthen from the right waist to the hip (the right side shortens due to the leg being raised) to equalize both sides of the body. Stay in the pose for several breaths and then lower the leg and repeat on the other side.

- *Supta Padangusthasana II* (FIGURE 13-15, p 172). Lie down and raise the right leg to perpendicular. Belt the arch of the foot and hold onto the belt with the right hand. Fully stretch the legs throughout the pose, unless this causes pain. Then allow the knee(s) to bend. On an exhalation, lower the right leg down to the right side. Avoid allowing the right hip to come up. The hips must remain level with each other, so the leg may not reach the floor. Keep the outer foot parallel to the floor. Avoid letting the leg move directly out to the side. Keep it higher than the hip. Look at the ceiling. Remain in the pose for a few breaths and then carefully raise the leg back up to the perpendicular, release the grasp of the hand and lower the leg to the floor. Repeat on the other side.

Lie down with the front on the floor and a folded blanket supporting the pelvic area. Put a weight of 9–11kg (20–25lb) on the hips so the buttocks are pressed down and away from each other (toward the floor). This releases the sciatic nerve.

Once the sharp pain of sciatica is decreased, the following postures can be performed regularly to lessen occurrence of sciatica. All standing postures should be practised against a wall or a counter for support and alignment. When turning to the right side in the pose, turn the right foot out more than 90°. The right heel may be placed on a support (a block or a lower book) so the sciatic nerve has room to stretch with comfort and ease.

- *Utthita Trikonasana* (FIGURES 10-4–10-6, p 108). Begin by standing in Tadasana. Walk your feet 1.2–1.4m (4ft–4ft 6in) apart and actively stretch your arms all the way from the heart to the fingertips. Feel the opening of the chest and the upper ribs as a result of the active stretch of the arms. Turn your left foot in 15° and revolve your right leg out. The right foot is at 110°–120° angle to the left foot, and the right and left heels are in line with each other. The right leg is the front leg, and the left leg is the back leg. Plant and spread your active yoga feet and lift the inner and outer arches up. Inhale, lengthening up through the legs and stretching them fully. Maintain the lifting of the kneecaps by contracting the quadriceps. Exhale. Elongate the sides of the body as you inhale and expand your lungs and spread the ribs. Exhale and extend laterally over your right leg, bending from the hip. Remember, it is not about how far you go down to the side; it's about being strong, extended and balanced while moving directly to the side over the right leg. This helps keep the pose in your legs so the spine can maintain its length and freedom. Place the right fingertips lightly on the right shin. Keep extending through both arms and equally through both sides of the body. Have the head in line with the spine, and lengthen from the crown of the head to the coccyx. Look straight ahead. Try to keep the back of the body in one plane. Frequently, the upper body is leaning forward of the lower body. Find the balance between ease and effort. Check your breathing. Is it ragged or held, indicating overexertion, or is it smooth and even, indicating ease? Maintain the pose for several breaths. See if you can continue elongating the body and opening the chest with every inhalation. Breathe normally. Inhale and come up out of the pose by grounding the feet and stretching up and back into your left hand. Release the arms to your sides, bring the feet to parallel, and walk back into Tadasana. Repeat on the other side.

- *Utthita Parsvakonasana* (FIGURE 10-12, p 114). In this posture, there is a long diagonal stretch on the upper side of the body, all the way from the foot to the fingertips. Start in Tadasana and jump or walk the legs wide apart to a comfortable distance (even wider than Trikonasana). Extend the arms out to the sides. Turn the left foot in 15° and revolve the right leg out. Heel is in line with heel. Ground the feet, spread the toes and lift the arches. Keeping the feet active, firm the muscles to the bone throughout the posture to keep the energy flowing, to support the knees and to maintain a stable base of the legs and feet. Inhale through the nostrils, infusing the body with the breath as though you were smelling a pleasing fragrance, and lengthen up through the legs and the sides of the body. This will lift and expand the chest. Exhale fully as you bend the right leg (at the hip, knee and ankle), with the knee in line with the heel. The leg will form a 90° angle. Bend the torso from the hips directly to the side over the right leg and bring the right hand behind the right foot, fingertips touching the ground. Turn the left arm up from the shoulder. Inhale and extend the left arm up and over the head. This external rotation of the left arm flattens the shoulder blade on the back and opens the chest. As you firm the outer edge of the left foot downward, lengthen up the left side of the body into the fingertips. Stretch into the fingertips and elongate both sides of the body evenly. Look straight ahead, with the chest facing forward, keeping the head in line with the spine, and observing the marvellous diagonal stretch you have created on the left side of the body. Stretch into the crown of the head and into the coccyx. Continue breathing naturally and smoothly. Elongate the right side from the hip to the armpit. Keep the shoulder blades on the back. Feel the opening and stretching of the pelvis. Stay in the pose for a few breaths. Enjoy this strong, dynamic stretch, moving past all limitations. Keep reaching. Come up out of the pose pressing into the right foot, lengthening the right leg, and reaching out the left arm. Turn the feet back to parallel and then repeat on the other side.

- *Ardha Chandrasana* (FIGURE 10-23, p 121). Stand in Tadasana. Walk your feet wide apart. Raise and extend the arms out to the sides. Turn the right foot in 15° and revolve the left leg out. Inhale from the legs and lift the ribs, and on the exhalation come into Trikonasana. Pause for a moment and enjoy the pose. Look forward throughout the pose, instead of turning the head to look down. Place your right hand on your hip and keep it there. As you reach out with your left hand, bend the left leg to a right angle and place the fingertips of the left hand firmly on the floor, several centimetres in front of the left toes. Draw your arm up into the shoulder socket from the cupping action of your fingertips. If your fingers do not reach the floor, use a block to bring the floor to you. Press into the left foot, stretch the leg fully, and draw the standing leg muscles up to the hip socket. At the same time, lift the right leg up parallel to the floor. Pull up the standing leg kneecap. Extend through the right heel and balls of the foot to maintain energy and firmness in the leg. Keep lengthening both sides of the body from the hips to the armpits, paying particular attention to the left side.

Stretch from the coccyx to the crown of the head. Look straight ahead and see if you can turn your body to face forwards. Firm the bottom hip under the top hip so the hips become stacked. Breathe! Root the left foot into the floor and stay in the pose for several breaths. See if you can extend your right arm up, palm facing forwards. Otherwise, keep the hand on the hip. Smile! Remember that this pose is called half moon. The moon gracefully appears and (seemingly) disappears from the sky so gracefully and effortlessly. It seems to float in the sky. Can you achieve this graceful floating quality in Ardha Chandrasana, using your breath to link with the movement for a flowing sequence in and out of the pose?

- *Tadasana* (FIGURE 10-1, p 104). Start by placing your feet hip distance apart. Turn the toes in slightly to keep the broadness of the lower back. Have your arms by your sides. When viewed from one side, the ear, shoulder, hip, knee and ankle should form a straight, vertical line. Create your yoga feet by spreading the toes and balls of the feet, pressing into the big and little toe mounds and the centre of the heel. Bring the weight a little more into the heels. Lift your arches as you ground the feet. Enhance this action by lengthening your leg muscles all the way up to your hips. Lift the top of the kneecaps up by contracting the quadricep muscle. Firm the muscles of the thigh to the bone. Now you have created a strong and stable base from which the torso will be able to extend. This is like creating the mantle for the mountain to rise out of. Place your hands on your hips and lift the sides of the body from your hips to your armpits. This action creates length and space in the spine. Bring your arms back to your sides without losing the lift of the spine, lengthen up through the crown of your head. Try to balance your head over the pelvis. Make sure the shoulders are relaxed and are not riding up to the ears. Press your shoulder blades into your back. Lift and broaden your chest. Breathe, remaining aware of how it feels to be in alignment.

- *Uttanasana* (FIGURE 10-34, p 127). Stand in Tadasana with feet hip-width apart, toes turned in slightly and heels turned out. Inhale , rooting down into the foundation of the feet and fully stretching up through the legs and the spine to the crown of the head. Roll the upper inner thighs and groin back, keeping the lower back broad. Draw the shoulder blades into the back to lift and open the chest. Maintain active yoga feet and a strong lift of the inner groin and legs. Actively lift and stretch your side ribs and spine up and over as you exhale and bend forwards, folding at the hips. Let the arms come down toward the floor. Place the fingertips on the floor in front of the feet. The legs draw up so the spine can release down. Breathe and allow the effects of gravity to release the back muscles and spine downwards. Contract the kneecaps and the quadricep muscle to help the hamstrings lengthen. Broaden the backs of the calves and the backs of the thighs. When you are ready to come up, press the feet down and keep the legs really active, so that the strength of the thigh muscles support the stretch of the hamstring. This will prevent the feeling of locking the knees (hyperextension of the knees, pressing the knees back). Look forward, lengthening the crown of the head and the coccyx away from each other. Inhale and come up with a concave back.

· *Ardha Uttanasana* (FIGURE 9-28, p 97). Place the hands on the wall at shoulder height and press the hands into the wall. As the hands root into the wall, the arms stretch back into the shoulder socket. Remember, for every action there is an equal and opposite reaction. The elbows are firm and straight. Continue lengthening from the shoulders to the buttock bones, making the sides of the waist long. Keep the shoulder blades in contact with the back body and back ribs. This stabilizes the shoulder joint and helps to open the chest. Even in a forward bend the chest remains open and the spine remains long. This action will help keep the spine happy, whereas the legs should do the pose so the spine receives the action. The body is parallel to the floor, with the head between the arms. The neck and head are in line with the rest of the spine. The crown of the head stretches to the wall as the coccyx lengthens to the middle of the room. The heels are in line with the buttock bones, and the feet are hip-width (or wider) apart. The toes are slightly turned in with the heels turned out. Tight hamstrings require a wider leg stance. Maintain active yoga feet and legs. The body is parallel to the floor. Make sure that you are not pressing the shoulders or front ribs down in an effort to open the body. You want a long line of stretch from the fingertips to the buttock bones and from the buttock bones to the heels. If the body hangs from a joint (shoulder, hyperextended knees, floating ribs), then the line of energy will be broken and the extension and stretch will occur in the tendons and ligaments instead of the muscles of the stomach. Broaden the lower back by spreading the buttock bones, letting the inner thighs hug the thighbones (away from each other). Pull the hips and the tops of the thighs back towards the middle of the room to create even more length in the spine. Feel the terrific space and length in the torso and the back of the legs. Stay for a few breaths and enjoy the space you have created in your body. The pose can also be done fully supported as a restorative pose, by resting the torso on a table.

· *Adho Mukha Svanasana* (FIGURE 9-32, p 99). Start on the hands and knees. Place the hands slightly forward of the shoulders and the knees under the hips. The inner arms face each other and the elbows are straight and firm. Let the shoulder blades come onto the back. Observe that the upper arm bones connect into the shoulder socket. Let the arms receive the weight of the upper body. The pelvis is in a neutral position, horizontal to the floor. Tuck the toes under. Plant the hands firmly on the floor and spread the fingers evenly apart. Press the palms, knuckles and fingers into the floor. Especially press down the index-finger knuckle and balance the weight on either side of the hand (just like we do for the feet in standing poses). These are important actions to maintain throughout the pose, as the hands are part of the pose's foundation, and they must stay rooted for extension of the spine to occur. Inhale and lift the hips and buttocks up and back, straighten the legs and, on the exhalation, let the head drop between the arms. Turn the toes in slightly and the heels out to broaden the lower back, soften the stomach and lengthen the groin. Relax the neck. Press the front of the thighs back to elongate the torso. Let the spine lengthen from the top of the head to the coccyx into one long line of extension. Press the heels down, but keep stretching the back of the legs up. The heels are stretching towards the floor. They might even make it to the floor, but do not force this action if it is not happening. Lift the shins out of the top of the ankles as you press the heels down. The feet are also working, spreading, grounding with arches lifting to enhance the upward extension of the legs. Fully stretch the legs, lift the kneecaps and firm the thighs. Stretch into your fingertips and press the entire hand down. Keeping this action, lengthen up through the arms to the buttock bones. Keep the arms as long as possible. Bending the elbows will make it difficult to transfer the weight of the body from the arms to the buttocks. Remain in the pose for several breaths, extending the spine on the inhalation and deepening into the pose and releasing unnecessary tension on the exhalation. Then bend the knees and come down.

    A fabulous way to practise downward-facing dog for sciatica and other lower back conditions is by pulling the hips back, either with the use of wall ropes, a belt looped around door handles or by having another person stand behind you and pull your hips back. This action creates traction on the spine and often provides relief from pain.

· *Bharadvajasana on a Chair* (FIGURE 12-1, p 156). Sit sideways on a chair. The left side of the body is next to the back of the chair. Plant your feet flat on the floor with heels under knees. If your feet do not make it to the floor, then bring the floor to you by placing a book or two under the feet. Hold onto the topsides of the chair back, bend the elbows and pull them apart to stretch and open the ribcage, making more room for the breath to enter. Press the buttock bones down into the chair seat as you inhale and lengthen the sides of the body. Exhale and gradually revolve the body around the spine towards the back of the chair. With every inhalation, create extension and space in the body. After three or four breaths, carefully unwind and return to the centre. Repeat on the other side.

· *Savasana* (FIGURE 18-1, p 241). Lie down on the floor with the knees bent. Place the back of the calves on the seat of a chair so that they are fully supported. The thighs are perpendicular to the floor. The head and neck can be lying on a folded blanket. Placing a 2.25 or 4.5kg (5 or 10lb) bag of rice or flour on the lower abdomen while in this position feels wonderful. The abdominal muscles soften and the lower-back muscles release and broaden. Stay in this pose for 5, 10 or 15 minutes, relaxing and softening.

Cancer

Eighty per cent of all illnesses are stress-related. It is chronic stress that tips the balance between ease and disease. In today's society, daily living has become very complex. A growing number of studies indicate that stress influences the immune system and affects the development and growth of diseases such as cancer and AIDS. People who have been given the diagnosis of cancer have many extra layers of stress added onto their baseline stress level.

A pivotal 1989 study, conducted by Stanford, USA, psychiatrist David Speigel, demonstrated that women with metastatic breast cancer who were in cancer support groups lived longer than those who were not. The experience of the support group seemed to provide protection against stress.

Many cancer trusts throughout the UK now believe that yoga can reduce levels of stress and bring about feelings of relaxation and well-being, and that they can enhance the quality of life for some patients with cancer. The British Wheel of Yoga (*www.bwy.org.uk*, see Appendix IV) maintains a register of teachers in all areas; New Approaches to Cancer (*www.anac.org.uk*) provides free information and advice on a wide range of complementary therapies, and maintains a register of yoga teachers throughout the UK; and the Yoga for Health Foundation offers courses of yoga for people with cancer (*www.yogaforhealthfoundation.co.uk*).

The diagnosis of cancer is frightening, isolating and anxiety-provoking. So many crucial decisions to be made in so little time. It may seem paradoxical that you can relax during this time of acute stress, but it is possible with yoga and meditation. The one-pointed focus of yoga allows the scattered, frazzled mind to concentrate on the present moment and its feelings and sensations. Then the overwhelming nature of reality can be managed, one step at a time.

Surgery, chemotherapy, radiation and medication all have a huge impact upon the entire person. Side effects such as sleep disturbances, pain, fatigue, nausea, flu-like symptoms and chemotherapy-induced menopause interfere with a person's well-being and daily functioning.

Yoga can help reduce these side effects and stress by working with the breath, awareness and movement. Breath and awareness are primary. Healing necessitates that we slow down the body and the mind, something that the system of yoga is designed to do beautifully. The asanas were developed to exercise every muscle, nerve and gland in the body, and as such, they bring about the release of blocked energy and tension. The organ systems (stomach, liver, kidneys, lungs, heart, small intestine, large intestine, spleen, pancreas and gall bladder) also benefit. They are stretched, toned, stimulated and massaged through the actions of the postures.

Gentle yoga postures that isolate muscle groups allow muscles to be comfortably stretched, while keeping the mind and the nervous system in the relaxation response. Active and restorative poses are beneficial. Breath with stretch is inspiring. It invites the breath in. Forward bends, backward bends, twists and mild inversions can help gently stretch tight muscles, fascia, scar tissue and discomfort resulting from surgery. A muscle worked in this way will be flexible when brought to its edge and soft while at rest.

The lymphatic system is designed to vacuum out the third spaces (between tissues) and pump waste back into the circulatory system for disposal. The 'pump' for the lymphatic system is the muscles. This underscores the importance of working the muscles; however, you do not want your muscles to be overly pumped. In aerobic and weight-lifting exercises, muscles stay contracted much longer after the workout is over than muscle that has been gently stretched and strengthened by yoga postures. This stresses the muscles and causes unnecessary fatigue. Contracted muscles consume more oxygen than relaxed muscles and use up oxygen vital for healing.

Movement should be synchronized with the breath. Yoga postures linked with the breath provide a strong grounding and centring vital to cancer patients who feel that their lives are out of their control. This centring process enables you to regain a sense of perspective and calm, as it brings you back into yourself at a very deep and quiet level.

A simple technique called three-part breathing, done lying down with bent legs, can be used as one example of the breath's healing benefits. Three-part breathing systematically brings the breath into the stomach, diaphragm and chest. This allows for a complete breath and increased lung capacity. With practice the exhalation can be maintained for twice as long as the inhalation. Amazingly, extending the exhalation twice as long as the inhalation creates seven times more oxygen circulating in the body than a shallow breath. (Please note that people experiencing depression are not advised to prolong their exhalations. Instead, it is recommended that these individuals lengthen the inhalation relative to the exhalation.)

Cancer cells proliferate in an oxygen-deprived (anaerobic) environment, so the increase in oxygen discourages the growth of new cancer cells. Blood alkalinity is also increased as a result of additional oxygen. The more alkaline the blood, the more resistant and stronger the immune system is to pathogens such as cancer.

The complete breath with the prolonged exhalation sends a message to the brain and the parasympathetic nervous system to begin the relaxation response. Heart rate decreases as the breath slows and deepens. Feelings of tension and stress diminish. Deep breathing also decreases thoracic pressure and increases lymphatic flow and drainage, vital to the body's ability to transport and expel waste. Another by-product is increased flexibility of the blood vessels so they can optimally expand and contract to circulate the blood effectively. (High blood pressure means your blood vessels have lost their ability to be flexible.)

The practice of yoga serves to heighten mind and body awareness. Focus on the present moment occurs during yoga postures, breathing exercises, relaxation techniques and guided meditation. These practices bring us into close, intimate contact with our sensations and feelings, and this can change our attitudes and how we deal with our relationship to cancer and healing.

After working consciously with the breath and yoga postures, it is time for deep relaxation. Guided relaxation and meditation with imagery have been found to be very effective for reducing pain, fatigue and stress. It is extremely replenishing and relaxing, and at the same also trains the mind to observe, focus and be non-judgmental. Meditation is an extremely important tool for people with cancer and other life- threatening illnesses. With the never-ending crucial decisions to be made during treatment for cancer, it is vital to maintain as much clarity of thought as possible. Meditation helps silence all the anxious and distracting voices inside the head.

This ability to discipline the mind positively affects an individual's perception of life. Illness can become an opportunity for self-discovery and growth. You can look at your illness as separate from your true self, rather than allowing yourself to be totally defined by the illness. Pain management through relaxation and meditation becomes possible as the body and mind lose their tight grip and surrender to the present reality.

Relaxation is the key to managing the stress and tension that accompany the experience of living with cancer. The discipline of yoga provides a potent arsenal of self-help tools. Working with breath, awareness and movement, yoga can guide the cancer patient through the healing process with as much ease and grace as possible.

More and more yoga teachers are being trained and have experience working with cancer patients. Any teacher who is sensitive to the needs of her students should be able to be aware of the needs of someone with cancer. The resource section at the end of the book lists organizations and reading material to help you find a good teacher or programme.

The message for cancer patients regarding exercise is this: honour your needs, take it easy, don't go all the way, find an inner place that is comfortable, watch your movements with awareness, and work isolated muscle groups in conjunction with the breath.

Multiple Sclerosis

Multiple sclerosis (MS) is an auto-immune disease in which the myelin sheath surrounding nerves in the brain and the spinal cord is destroyed. As a result, the transmission of nerve impulses from the body to the brain is impaired. Symptoms of MS can include:

· Numbness and tingling in the extremities
· Weakness
· Lack of co-ordination
· Difficulty with balance and gait
· Slurring of speech
· Impaired vision
· Tremors
· Bladder and bowel dysfunction
· Vertigo
· Sensitivity to heat
· Paralysis
· Pain

In time, secondary symptoms such as poor posture, alignment, trunk control, muscle imbalances, decreased bone density,and shallow and inefficient breathing occur. The illness may also lead to job loss, disruption of important relationships and depression.

Yoga has become a recognized way of managing MS symptoms. The combination of yoga postures, br eathing exercises, relaxation techniques and meditation serve to:

· Heighten body-mind awareness
· Release muscular tension
· Decrease muscle spasticity
· Improve balance and co-ordination
· Increase flexibility
· Increase strength
· Reduce fatigue
· Improve circulation

- Improve breathing
- Improve organ function
- Increase the ability to manage stress
- Enhance feelings of well-being
- Increase energy and vitality

Breath is the key to opening the body. All movement is done in conjunction with the breath. It is important for individuals with MS not to become overheated or tired. Less is more here. Rest is essential. Guided imagery and mindfulness-based meditation are extremely valuable for reducing stress and calming the mind and the emotions.

If you're able to stand with steadiness and stability, standing poses – such as Trikonasana (FIGURE 10-4, p 108), Virabhadrasana I (FIGURE 10-10, p 112), Virabhadrasana II (FIGURE 10-18, p 118) and Ardha Uttanasana (FIGURE 9-28, p 97) – can be done with the support of the wall or a counter. The standing poses may also be done with chairs.

Seated poses on the floor with wall support–such as Baddha Konasana (FIGURE 11-18, p 143), Upavistha Konasana (FIGURES 11-36 and 11-37, p 152) and Janu Sirsasana (FIGURE 11-26, p 147) – are also beneficial. Gentle seated poses in a chair, such as turning the head from side to side (co-ordinated with breath) and dropping the chin to chest, are excellent for neck and shoulder mobility. Single- and double-arm raises, inhaling up and exhaling down, open the chest and lungs and ease shoulder flexibility. Bending forward from the hips lengthens the spine and the back side of the body. Placing the hands on the sides of the chair and lifting the heart creates back-bending action in the upper back and opens the chest for fuller breathing. Circling shoulders, wrists and ankles, wiggling the fingers and the toes, helps circulation and joint mobility. Seated knee-to-chest and leg raises develop strength and flexibility.

Supported, restorative poses – such as Supta Baddha Konasana (FIGURE 13-1, p 163), Viparita Karani (FIGURE 14-14, p 204), and Supported Savasana (FIGURE 18-1, p 241) – are essential to soothe the nervous system and open the lungs. Drinking lots of water is also vital to replenish and recharge, as well as fight against constipation and sluggish digestion.

Simple lying-down postures – such as single knee to chest and modified Supta Padangusthasana (FIGURE 13-11, p 170) – help release the lower back and the hamstrings. Observing the natural breath, practising three-part breathing and lengthening the exhalation without strain all serve to improve energy flow and circulation. Relaxation and meditation replenish energy and train the mind to let go and accept the present moment.

Basic Yoga Poses

T his appendix lists the basic yoga poses in Sanskrit, along with their English translations.

Adho Mukha Svanasana: downward-facing dog

Anantasana: serpent pose

Ardha Chandrasana: half moon pose

Ardha Uttanasana: half-forward standing bend

Baddha Konasana: cobbler pose

Balasana: child's pose

Bharadvajasana on Chair: sage twist

Bhujangasana: cobra pose

Chattaranga Dandasana: four-limbed staff pose

Dandasana: staff or rod pose

Garudasana: eagle pose

Gomukhasana: cow's head pose

Halasana: plough pose

Janu Sirsasana: head-to-knee pose

Jathara Parivartanasana: stomach-turning pose

Maricyasana III: sage twist

Navasana: boat pose

Parivritta Parsvakonasana: revolved extended side-angle pose

Parivritta Trikonasana: revolved triangle

Parsva Upavistha Konasana: sideways wide-angle pose

Parsvottanasana: sideways extended pose

Parvatasana: seated mountain pose

Paschimottanasana: seated straight-leg forward bend

Prasarita Padottanasana: wide-legged forward bend

Salabhasana: locust pose

Salamba Sarvangasana: shoulderstand

Savasana: basic relaxation pose

Setu Bandha Sarvangasana: bridge pose

Sirsasana: headstand

Standing Maricyasana: sage twist on a chair

Sukhasana: easy pose

Supta Baddha Konasana: supported cobbler pose

Supta Padangusthasana: reclining hand on the big toe pose

Supta Virasana: reclining hero pose

Surya Namaskar: sun salutation

Tadasana: mountain pose

Triang Mukhaikapada Paschimottanasana: half virasana forward bend

Upavistha Konasana: seated wide-angle pose

Urdhva Mukha Svanasana: upward-facing dog

Urdhva Prasarita Padasana: upward spread-out foot pose

Utkatasana: chair pose or fierce warrior

Uttanasana: standing forward bend

Utthita Hasta Padangusthasana: extended hand on the foot posture

Utthita Parsvakonasana: extended side-angle pose

Utthita Trikonasana: extended triangle pose

Vajrasana: thunderbolt pose

Vasisthasana: one-arm side balance pose

Viparita Dandasana: inverted staff pose

Viparita Karani: supported legs up the wall pose

Virabhadrasana I, II, III: warrior pose

Virasana: hero's pose

Vrksasana: tree pose

Yoga Glossary for Poses

The Sanskrit names of poses can be confusing and even intimidating for beginners of yoga. Asana means 'pose' and is the suffix for all poses. Sanskrit is a systematic and phonetically based language. There are suffixes and prefixes of words that always have the same meaning. Learning the Sanskrit names of the poses helps to understand yoga.

adho: downwards
ananta: infinite, the name of a serpent
ardha: half
baddha: bound
bala: child
chandra: moon
danda: a staff
eka pada: one leg
garuda: eagle
gomukha: a face resembling a cow, narrow at one end and broad at the other end
hala: a plough
hasta: the hand
hatha: forcibly or against one's will; a discipline
janu: the knee
jathara: the stomach or abdomen
kona: angle
Marichi: the name of a sage
mukha: face
pada: foot
padangustha: big toe
parivartana: turning around, revolving
parivritta: turned around, revolved
parsva: the side, lateral
paschima: West; the back side of the body
paschimottana: intense stretch of the back side of the body
pincha: the chin, a feather
prana: breath, respiration, life force, vital energy
prasarita: spread out, stretched out
raja-kapota: king pigeon
salabha: locust
sarvanga: the whole body

setu: a bridge
setu bandha: the construction of a bridge
sirsa: the head
sukha: happiness, joy
supta: lying down
surya: the sun
tada: a mountain
tri: three
trianga: three limbs
trikona: a triangle
upavistha: seated
urdhva: raised, upwards
urdhva mukha: upward-facing
utkata: powerful, fierce
uttana: an intense stretch
utthita: raised up, extended, stretched
vajra: a thunderbolt
Vasistha: a celebrated sage
viparita: inverted, reversed
vira: a hero, brave
Virabhadra: a powerful hero or warrior
vrksa: tree

Bibliography

This appendix will provide you with a 'futher readings' list, should you be interested in learning more about various types of yoga, its history and its masters.

◎ Anderson, Sandra and Rolf Sovik, Psy.D. *Yoga: Mastering the Basics.* (The Himalayan Institute Press, 2000).

◎ Austin, Miriam. *Yoga for Wimps.* (Sterling Publishing Co., Inc., 2000).

◎ Balaskas, Janet. *Preparing for Birth with Yoga.* (Element Books, 1994).

◎ Boucher, Sandy. 'Yoga for Cancer'. *Yoga Journal,* May–June 1999, pp 42–49, 135–138.

◎ Browning Miller, Elise and Blackman. 'Six Stretches to Do at your Desk'.*Yoga Journal,* March–April 1999.

◎ Browning Miller, Elise. 'Yoga for Scoliosis'. *The Spinal Connection,* National Scoliosis Foundation, 1997.

◎ Bruyere, Rosalyn L. and Jeanne Farrens. *Wheels of Light, A Study of the Chakras, Volume I.* (Bon Productions, 1989).

◎ *Journal's Yoga Basics: The Essential Beginner's Guide to Yoga for a Lifetime of Health and Fitness.* (Henry Holt and Company, 1997).

◎ Cope, Stephen. *Yoga and the Quest for the True Self.* (Bantam Books, 1999).

◎ Devi, Nischala Joy. *The Healing Path of Yoga: Time-Honored Wisdom and Scientifically Proven Methods That Alleviate Stress, Open Your Heart, and Enrich Your Life.* (Three Rivers Press, 2000).

◎ Desikachar,T.K.V. *The Heart of Yoga: Developing a Personal Practice.* (Inner Traditions International, 1995).

◎ Dworkis, Sam. *Recovery Yoga, A Practical Guide for Chronically Ill, Injured, and Post-Operative People.* (Three Rivers Press, 1997).

◎ Feuerstein, Georg, Ph.D. 'A Short History of Yoga', 2000. Downloaded from AOL, 8 January, 2001.

◎ Feuerstein, Georg, Ph.D. *The Shambala Encyclopedia of Yoga.* (Allen Unwin, 1997).

◎ Feuerstein, Georg, Ph.D. and Payne, Ph.D. *Yoga For Dummies.* (Hungry Minds, Inc.).

◎ Hammond, Holly. 'Meet the Innovators!' *Yoga Journal,* October 2000, pp 81–89.

◎ Iyengar, B.K.S. *Yoga, The Path to Holistic Health.* (Dorling Kindersley, 2001).

◎ Iyengar, B.K.S. *The Tree of Yoga.* (HarperCollins, 1988).

◎ Iyengar, B.K.S. *Light on Pranayama.* (HarperCollins, 1994).

◎ Iyengar, B.K.S. *Light On Yoga.* (HarperCollins, 1976).

◎ Iyengar, Geeta S. *Yoga A Gem for Women.* (Timeless Books, 1990).

◎ Jordan, Sandra. *Yoga for Pregnancy.* (St. Martin's Press, 1987).

◎ Lasater, Judith, Ph.D., P.T. *Relax and Renew, Restful Yoga for Stressful Times.* (Rodmell Press, 1995).

◎ Maddern, Jan. *Yoga Builds Bones.* (Element Books, 2000).

◎ Mehta, Silva, Mira, and Shyam. *Yoga The Iyengar Way.* (Dorling Kindersley, 1990).

◎ Raman, Krishna, M.D. *A Matter of Health, Integration of Yoga and Western Medicine for Prevention and Cure.* (Eastwest Books Pvt. Lmt., 1998).

◎ Scaravelli, Vanda. *Awakening the Spine.* (HarperCollins, 1991).

◎ Schatz, Mary Pullig, M.D. *Back Care Basics, A Doctor's Gentle Yoga Program for Back and Neck Pain Relief.* (Berkeley, California, 1992).

◎ Shearer, Alistair. *Effortless Being: The Yoga Sutras of Patanjali.* (Mandala Books, 1980).

◎ Sivananda Yoga Vedantic Centre. *Yoga Mind and Body.* (Dorling Kindersley, 2000).

◎ Stiles, Mukunda. *Structural Yoga Therapy, Adapting to the Individual.* (Samuel Weiser, Inc., 2000).

◎ Todd, Mabel E. *The Thinking Body.* (Dance Horizons/Princeton Book Co., 1937).

Resources

I n this appendix, you'll find numerous resources to augment the information in this book. From magazines to Web sites, this appendix has it all.

Yoga Magazines

In addition to providing great information on yoga, the following magazines publish annual updates of their yoga teachers directories. These directories include teachers in countries throughout the world.

◎ *Spectrum*
The British Wheel of Yoga
25 Jermyn Street
Sleaford NG34 7RU
Phone: 01529-306851
Web site: *www.bwy.org.uk*

◎ *Yoga and Health*
Yoga Today, Ltd
PO Box 29
Brighton BN1 8JQ
Phone: 01273-563111
Web site: *www.yogaandhealthmag.co.uk*

◎ *Yoga Journal*
2054 University Avenue
Berkeley, California 94704, USA
Phone: 00 1 510-841-9200
Web site: *www.yogajournal.com*

◎ *Yoga International*
RR 1, Box 407
Honesdale, Pennsylvania, USA
Phone: 00 1 570-253-4929
Web site: *www.yimag.com*

◎ *Yoga Magazine*
319 Bethnal Green Road
London E2 6AH
Phone: 020-7729-5454
Web site: *www.yogamagazine.co.uk*

Different Styles of Yoga

There are many different styles of yoga. The following is a list of organizations for you to turn to if you want to find out more. They can help you find a yoga class or teacher near you, and can advise on yoga videos and equipment and clothing.

◎ The British Wheel of Yoga
25 Jermyn Street
Sleaford NG34 7RU
Phone: 01529-306851
Web site: *www.bwy.org.uk*

◎ Iyengar Yoga Institute
223a Randolph Avenue
London W9 1NL
Phone: 020-7264-3080
Web site: *www.iyi.org.uk*

◎ Yoga for Health Foundation
Ickwell Bury
Ickwell
Biggleswade SG18 9EF
Phone: 01767 627271
Web site: *www.yogaforhealthfoundation.co.uk*

◎ Yoga Scotland
Web site: *www.yogascotland.org.uk*

◎ Yoga Therapy Centre
Web site: *www.yogatherapy.org*

◎ Yoga Directory
Web site: *www.yogadirectory.com*

Model Biographies

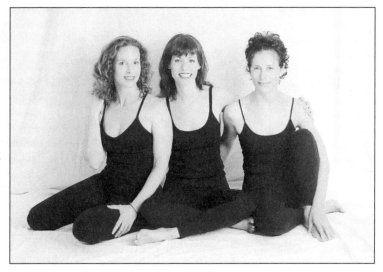

The models (left to right): Mary Sinclair, Cynthia Worby and Monica Beatriz

Mary Sinclair

Mary Sinclair (left) has been practicing yoga for 21 years and is certified to teach in the Iyengar tradition. She has also studied in India several times. Mary's emphasis is on having fun while developing alignment and gaining flexibility through strength and balance. She is a massage therapist in Connecticut, USA.

Cynthia Worby

Cynthia Worby (centre) has been practising yoga for 12 years. Her training has been in Iyengar Yoga and Ashtanga Yoga. She has studied with many wonderful teachers and continues to do so. Her teaching style emphasizes learning how to do the poses correctly with a balance between ease and effort, while listening to and honouring the body. She has been the director of Bedford Yoga in Bedford, New York, USA, for the past 10 years, and she was the president of the Yoga Teachers Association of Westchester County and the surrounding Metropolitan New York area for three years. Cynthia has taught workshops for yoga students and teachers, children and pre-teens, and people of all ages. She has appeared on local radio and television programs speaking about the many benefits of yoga. Cynthia has a Master's degree in Social Work and a Master's degree in Public Health.

Monica Beatriz

Monica Beatriz (right) is an enthusiastic student of yoga. Her background in architecture, her personal practice, as well as inspiring teachers, infuses insight into her classes, which integrate the principles of alignment with the transformational and philosophical aspects of yoga. She lives and teaches in Nyack, New York, USA.

Index